Prais

"*The Mother Load* is an honest and vulnerable journey through motherhood and mental health with your passionate guide, Meredith Ethington. Meredith is that friend who will sit you down and ask, 'How are you?' and actually listen because she doesn't want any mother to carry her load alone."

—Jen Mann, *New York Times* bestselling
author *Midlife Bites: Anyone Else
Falling Apart, Or Is It Just Me?*

"You know that person you call when everything is terrible, and you need the honest-to-God truth about what to do next? That's Meredith—and that is what this book is. Mer's writing often has me wondering if she is watching me. How does she KNOW? That's what Meredith's writing does best. Makes all of us feel a little less crazy, and a whole lot less alone."

—Mary Katherine Backstrom, bestselling
author of *Holy Hot Mess* and *Crazy Joy*

"Like Meredith, and pretty much every mom out there, I, too, have often wondered if I would survive the daily grind without losing my ever-loving mind. She sums it up perfectly in this book and made me feel seen. Meredith had me laughing and nodding repeatedly as I saw my own story in hers."

Kate Swenson, author of *Forever Boy:
A Mother's Memoir of Autism and Finding Joy*

"All moms—no matter if you're new to the game or not—need validation. Meredith provides that validation with a whopping dose of humor and honesty. Pick up this book when you need a moment to laugh, to nod in agreement or just need a few moments to feel seen and heard."

—Kate Auletta, Editor in Chief of Scary Mommy

"The *Mother Load* is the combination we all need of laughter with your best girlfriends and solidarity from someone who has been where you are. Meredith nails it once again with her witty, relatable, moving reflection on motherhood and mental illness."

—Sara Farrell Baker, Writer

"Real. Raw. Laugh-out-loud funny. Motherhood is awesome—and awful. Meredith isn't afraid to talk about both. You'll feel so seen. Finally."

—Robyn Gobbel, MSW

THE MOTHER LOAD

Surviving the Daily Grind *Without* Losing Your Ever-Loving Mind

MEREDITH ETHINGTON

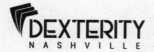

DEXTERITY
NASHVILLE

DEDICATION

For all the mothers fighting battles no one sees.

. . .

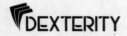

Dexterity, LLC
604 Magnolia Lane
Nashville, TN 37211

Printed in the United States of America.

First edition: 2023
10 9 8 7 6 5 4 3 2 1

ISBN: 9781947297647
ISBN: 9781947297654 (E-book)
ISBN: 9781947297661 (Audiobook)

Publisher's Cataloging-in-Publication Data

Names: Ethington, Meredith, author.
Title: The mother load : surviving the daily grind without losing your ever loving mind / Meredith Ethington.
Description: Includes bibliographical references. | Nashville, TN: Dexterity, 2023.
Identifiers: ISBN: 9781947297647 (hardcover) | 9781947297654 (ebook) | 9781947297661 (audio)
Subjects: LCSH Motherhood. | Mothers--Anecdotes. | Parenting. | Women--Humor. | Humorous stories.
| BISAC FAMILY & RELATIONSHIPS / Parenting / Motherhood
Classification: LCC HQ759 .E84 2023| DDC 306.8/743--dc23

Cover design by twoline STUDIO
Interior design by PerfecType, Nashville, TN

CONTENTS

CONTENTS

SECTION THREE
TOXIC POSITIVITY

SECTION FOUR
MENTAL ILLNESS

CONTENTS

INTRODUCTION

I'll never forget watching *Oprah* and listening to an expert say that the female brain shrinks by 8 percent during pregnancy. Is the 8 percent shrinkage permanent? Is it 8 percent with each child?

I joke with my husband that my brain has three times the shrinkage because I have three kids (if that's the way it works), which explains my "mom brain" tendencies. That is why I can't remember things and why I can't handle stressors in my life. It explains why I battle sensory overload all the time.

In my friend circle, we all laugh off mom brain, but I have found my brain is different than the brain of my friends who have not had children.

And I don't believe it's as simple as our brain shrinking.

The pressure on moms today is unrelenting. We deal with keeping up with other mothers online; we deal with unwanted comments on how motherhood today "should" be. We face an overwhelming mental load to keep up with all the demands required of a woman to work, be a mom, and "have it all." And some of us—probably most of us—also struggle with mental illness.

Whether it is a temporary bout of postpartum depression, feeling overwhelmed from the pressures and expectations of modern society, or full-blown anxiety and depression, it seems like very few mothers in my circle remain unscathed by the changes that their brains go through while mothering.

It seems to me that most mothers experience mental health changes in one form or another.

Becoming a new mom is a lot to experience. I can attest that even mature motherhood is hard too. This mama's brain is worn out thanks to the seemingly endless loop it runs on.

I picture my tired mom brain a lot like that little brain cartoon with the arms and legs running. Have you seen that one?

Picture the mother load a lot like your mom brain— except your cute little mom brain signed up for a spin class that you weren't quite ready for. You go full speed while the music is pumping until suddenly you realize you must dart out and puke in the hallway trashcan.

The mother load can feel just like that.

I'm here to tell you that if you've got your pre-baby body back but not your pre-baby mind, you're not alone. And if you didn't get either your mind or body back, I'm right there with you.

As you read this book, I hope you'll realize your thoughts, feelings, and struggles surrounding motherhood are perfectly normal. That, yes, despite the glorious moments that come with being a mom, this is hard . . . for all of us. But as you navigate the following pages, I also hope you'll come to see the beauty that comes with loving and accepting your new reality—mom brain and all.

SECTION ONE

What Is the Mother Load?

It's not motherhood we want a break from, it's everything else we need to have a break from that distracts us from just being able to chill and enjoy motherhood. **—Laura Mazza**

CHAPTER 1

This Is Your Brain on Motherhood

Some of us were functioning as single adults and then crumpled after motherhood—which, when you think about it, makes a lot of sense. There is so much to worry about. So many complex decisions to make. So much to do.

And yes, we all fantasize about escaping to a deserted island after we become mothers.

The mental load we carry as mothers is so heavy, we dream about being alone so we don't have to worry about anyone else. We can't even go to the bathroom alone!

Can you imagine sitting by yourself with zero thoughts about your kids floating into your brain? Yeah—me neither.

Perhaps fantasizing about being alone is our brain's way of trying to protect us from the perceived or even real dangers of life. It's probably because we are terrified of screwing up. Or maybe we can't stand the thought of our kids experiencing real-life disappointments. It's heart-wrenching to think about the cruelty in the world that directly affects our children.

There's a lot to worry about as a mom, so we imagine alone time and kid-free thoughts because the scary thoughts that creep in feel like a load that we can't bear alone.

Post-Baby Body

The connection a mother has with her child places a weight on her shoulders because she can see every possible outcome. Show me a mom who's not afraid she'll emotionally scar her children for life. Show me a mom who isn't terrified she'll probably need therapy, despite her very best efforts not to screw up. The struggle is real. Oh, and let's talk about how the body changes along with the mind.

When I had my first baby, I was shocked at the ways my body changed, especially when I was nursing and my breasts became giant milk jugs squirting liquid all the time. My pelvic floor is undoubtedly ruined (yes, I know about Kegels). Our bodies go through enormous (pun intended) changes when we are pregnant, and I swear that after my first pregnancy, I could never drink room-temperature water again. In fact, the more ice the better.

Some of us never get our bodies back. My mother always talked about my great birthing hips, so I'm pretty sure I have had these same thighs since about age five.

Some women bounce back, and that is wonderful. No hard feelings. I'm not one of those women. I'm not one who can nurse for fourteen months and watch the weight fall off. I'm one of those women who can nurse for fourteen months and keep my nice plump, round, squishy figure to make that nutritious milk for my babies.

I never even attempted to lose those last fifteen pounds because I gained forty-five pounds when pregnant. I didn't necessarily give up on life either; I just accepted my mom bod. Why shouldn't we? Dads do.

I've learned to accept a lot of things that come with being a mom, but what I've had a hard time reconciling is the fact that my mind has never been the same. All the things that come with motherhood and the mental load was almost too much from the very beginning.

Post-Baby Mind

Our mind changes when we have kids. In fact, experts have barely scratched the surface of research on how much the mom brain changes after birth.

According to the expert on *Oprah*, we *know* that the brain is altered by motherhood. But how often do we really talk about how it may be permanently changed?

Is it possible that the mom brain makes us the real superheroes?

Women are predisposed to fight for their children from the moment they are born. Have you ever heard a mom say, "Don't make me pull out the bear claws"? She will turn into a mama bear in no time flat if someone is threatening her child. Moms have been this way since the beginning of time.

In 2020, a group of scientists found some fossil footprints, thousands of years old, that showed evidence that a woman was carrying a child as they ran from a giant predator. Most likely a giant sloth or a mammoth was on her tail. Her fight-or-flight instincts had to kick in as she scooped up her child and ran.

Luckily, we aren't escaping too many prehistoric predators these days, but parents in this century have plenty of other dangers and distractions. We have to worry about so much in order to protect our kids. I have stories—so many stories—that have tested my superhero theory.

When my youngest was about a year and a half and tumbling around like a sugared-up honey badger, I had an incident that goes down in hilarious infamy in our family.

I had one of those horrific nights when the colicky toddler with stomach issues was up every hour and I still had to get kids off to school. My three-year-old told me he changed his underwear when he woke up because "it was wet." It was laundry day anyway.

It's all good, Meredith. You've got this.

My oldest was finally off to kindergarten and I gathered a few extra things to take a load of laundry to the basement. I slipped through the door at the top of the stairs, trying to keep the devil cat (who recently tried to dine on my toddler's face) from running upstairs, where I was leaving the toddler for just a hot minute.

I tried to navigate the slippery tile death stairs with an annoying cat under my feet, when suddenly the cat attacked me (she smelled my weakened state) and I became the prey.

With a deep, aching soul sigh I headed back upstairs to bandage my bleeding leg.

I was so tired from the night before that I felt like crawling into any quiet, kid-less corner and rocking myself to sleep. I got my three-year-old out the door to a friend's house for a playdate, and I was starting to feel a little bit more like I had things under control.

"I am superwoman. Yes, I am. Yes, she is." I hear Alicia Keyes singing.

But laundry doesn't care if you feel like you've got it together. Laundry will humble you real quickly, and the loud buzzer from downstairs reminded me it was time to switch it.

I headed back to that door that leads to the death stairs. I kept it closed at all times to avoid my toddler from toddling downstairs to a hospital visit.

I headed back upstairs with a load in my arms and went to open the door at the top of the stairs leading into the kitchen, where my toddler was, but to my horror, it was locked.

Now, usually, you are grateful when your child reaches a new milestone—like mastering the pincer grasp—until he does something like lock you in the basement with a load of laundry in your arms.

Luckily, I had my cell phone in my pocket. I calmly called my husband and explained my dilemma.

He repeated back to me, "The baby locked you out?"

I heard laughter in the background.

"Are your coworkers laughing at me?"

He laughed. "They are saying, 'Child anarchy!'"

Clearly, I didn't see the humor, and I hung up the phone

trying to think of how I would get back inside before he started flushing valuables down the toilet.

I went outside. It was thirty-three degrees with a blizzard-like wind blowing. I had no shoes or coat, but my husband had suggested that I see if the front door was unlocked. It wasn't.

He also reminded me that the kids' window was probably still open from last night when we cracked it. Lovely. I get to shimmy all this booty through a barely cracked window. I knew the window was my only hope. Great. This was going to be awesome.

I went to the back deck and looked at the window. It was just high enough to be pull-up height. I haven't attempted a pull-up since the Presidential Physical Fitness Test in gym class. Hoisting myself up into it was not an option.

I looked around for something to climb on. I tried the sun-faded plastic patio chair, but it was too short.

Then I pictured my best bet: the eleven-year-old rusty, rickety grill. I heaved myself up on top, which was a reminder that becoming a cat burglar would never be a feasible career path for me. Really, any line of work that requires you to be alert, well-rested, and agile, and to have shoes on outdoors in the dead of winter.

Thank goodness I'm climbing in the back window where no one can see me. The last thing I need is a visit from the cops.

The window opened just enough that I had to make myself into a Flat Stanley and slide myself in.

And because kids can sometimes be little b-holes, the toddler started pointing at the window and laughing.

Real funny, kid. *Real* funny.

In that moment when I slid through a window not made for postpartum thighs, I thought of myself as Super Mom. After all, I can leap tiny grills and pull my post-baby butt through windows after my baby locks me out.

You need *skills* for that.

While we may not always need to be climbing through windows with our Spidey-senses on full alert, we have plenty of dangers to worry about. Not to mention important events we're expected to remember as we teach our kids, run a household, and hold down a job outside the home. No wonder the mental load moms carry is so draining.

We have to remember all of our stuff, all of our kids' stuff, and often the stuff our partner doesn't remember because of that pesky little selective hearing issue he has going on.

We can daydream all day long about how it would be nice to have that pre-baby mind back that didn't worry incessantly about all the things. We could make decisions about ourselves and no one else. And it would be so nice to not have the responsibilities of an entire household of people swimming in our heads. It would be so nice not to worry about the toddler falling downstairs or locking you out of your own home. We would be like the fun aunt all the time who could give out lollipops and ice cream and not worry about whether the kids would eat their dinner or what time they had to go to bed.

The to-do lists flooding your mind are normal on one hand because every woman struggles with the mental load of motherhood. But those lists are bound to take a toll if we don't farm out responsibilities, empty our brains, and give ourselves quiet moments to rest inside our own minds. At some point, we have to stop dreaming about the plan to escape to a deserted island with no responsibilities, and instead learn to cope with our new brains and the mental load that they now carry.

The mom brain gets a bad rap. It isn't a bad thing, it's just a new thing when you become a mom. Yes, it's tiring, and I can't keep up in spin class. It feels like a lot, and it is. But it's manageable with this incredible, Spidey-sense mom brain we have now that's thinking and worrying about all the things because we love our people.

We Can't Escape the Mental Load, but We Can Do Things to Help It

Here are some mental break ideas:

Shut down your mom brain.
Do your best to shut down your mom brain at the end of the day in a way that is healthy. Call me weird, but I love my mystery shows at the end of a long day. Give me an unsolved mystery from 1988, and I've forgotten all about the to-do list.

Connect with your partner in new ways.
Reconnect with your partner. You're parents with new responsibilities you didn't have before. This means carving out quality time. You can also try a brain dump session with

your partner and figure out what you can do together to help lighten the load.

Take breaks.

Allow yourself space from your children so you can recharge. Lightening the mental load depends on taking the time you need to find your center, catch your breath, and treat yourself to a latte or a glass of wine with a friend. Just slow down.

Don't forget who you are without kids.

How do we zero in on what makes us a unique person separate from our children? What makes us happy? What brings us joy outside of our little people? What will you do when they are gone? Because believe it or not, they do grow up.

> Lightening the mental load depends on taking the time you need to find your center, catch your breath, and treat yourself to a latte or a glass of wine with a friend. Just slow down.

The Mom Brain Has Superpowers

Mom brain makes us forget. Mom brain is tired, overworked, stressed, and, yes, even depressed and anxious.

We have to realize that the mom brain has superpowers. We can multitask like a boss, cooking dinner while helping a kid tie a shoe and nursing a baby who's strapped to us.

We have an infinite capacity to love like never before. We can shimmy ourselves through windows to save our toddlers from certain death.

We can have 384 imaginary tabs open and prioritize what needs to get our attention next.

Our brains can empathize with another human being like never before. Their pain is our pain. And it's magical to be able to be that person for another human. The mental load—dare I say it—is worth it.

The mom brain is our superpower, but it also needs to be nurtured and cared for. It needs a freaking break. It needs someone else to carry the load, or at least validate that load.

So yes, I would love to have that pre-baby mind back that could always remember where she last left her keys and didn't call her dog by one of her kids' names, but I wouldn't trade it for the parts of my brain that have been strengthened through motherhood.

If you stop and think about it, although our brains have changed permanently, they have superpowers they didn't have before. And those powers are going to help us.

"It's a scary thing for people. We don't know a lot about the brain and don't want to think that it might not go back," Dr. Cindy Barha said. *"But it doesn't need to go back. It shouldn't go back because it's changed. It's evolved."*

CHAPTER 2

For Better or . . . *Worse*?

I've told my husband on more than one occasion that I wish he could just peek into my brain for a day. I want him to see it. Feel what it's like to be me. I want him to experience the constant stream of consciousness that is full of tasks, checklists, and things I'm constantly willing myself to remember.

I want him to understand how hard I try to keep it all together, only to feel crushed when I forget something important because I had too much going on in my head. Too much to remember.

I don't want my husband to see my mental load to make him feel guilty. I want him to see the load so he'll understand me better.

You see, there are days when I can't relax like I want. My brain won't quit when I need it to. I can't seem to shake the damn mental load, and my husband doesn't seem to have it at all.

How is this fair?

For me, the mental load looks something like this (repeat all day long times infinity):

Do we have enough bread for lunch tomorrow?
I need to have a talk with the five-year-old about honesty and have him return that toy he "borrowed."
I hope I can get some sleep tonight. Like, actual real sleep where I have a dream or twitch or something. I should buy a sleep mask.
Did I put the laundry in the dryer?
How is the ceiling fan that dusty? Why is there so much dust on a fan that spins all day? How is that even possible?
I should wash our sheets. I bet Karen washes her sheets every week.
I need a freaking vacation from mom life, but who would remember that we need more ramen noodles?

My husband's thoughts after a long day of work? *I think I'll take a nap.*

I shared a picture of him resting on the sofa with these same sentiments on my Facebook page a few years ago and was surprised to see how many men came out to tell me how stereotypical I was being.

My husband works hard for our family. He provides and still comes home and helps with dinner, bedtime, and bills after a long hard day.

He's willing to do whatever needs to be done, but he just doesn't see it or care about it to the extent that I do. After twenty years of marriage, I'm learning to accept that.

When it's bothering me, I speak up. And when I do, he is the first to jump in and help.

Do Men Have a Mental Load?

It needs to be said: some men carry a heavy mental load. Depending on how you were raised and the responsibilities you grew up seeing as normal, anyone can carry a mental load. Including men.

My man carries a mental load for sure. He feels stressed about work and the load to support a family. He worries about the kids, and he stresses about how we are raising them.

The difference is that men often carry this mental load in silence, so we don't realize they actually have one.

Despite the mental weight men tend to bear in silence, research shows that it's the women who usually become weighed down by the mental load.

A 2019 study of heterosexual couples found that the women in the relationships tend to take on a significant amount of cognitive labor. They found this particularly true when it came to anticipating the needs of others and monitoring progress.[1]

Another study,[2] of mostly employed women, found that 88 percent of working women also reported they primarily managed routines at home, and 76 percent said they were mostly responsible for maintaining regular household standards and order.

Research suggests that same-sex couples seem to share the mental load more evenly. I can't help but think

17

it's totally possible for a heterosexual couple to have the same success.

So why is it that women tend to automatically assume the weight of the mental load and become overwhelmed by it all?

When we lost 8 percent of our brain with each kid, did that make extra room? Is that why we take on more of the household duties and always have 384 tabs open in our brains? Does that make room for that extra mental load?

Yes, it would be nice if my husband would be bothered by the same pencil that has been lying on the kitchen floor the same way I was bothered by it. But I wonder, would it really? I'm still not sure.

In my house, anyway, it balances out the family dynamic to have someone who isn't bothered by it. Because otherwise, we'd both be yelling at the kids constantly and in a constant state of annoyance.

Would I like it if he cared more so he would be more motivated the same way I am? Sure.

The mental load we carry as women is not the fault of our partners. But they can absolutely be the solution.

As we have evolved in our marriage, I've noticed a shift. He is bothered by the fact that I'm bothered. And he sincerely wants to help.

It makes me feel good when I say that we need to all spend fifteen minutes cleaning up, and he rallies the troops and we work together as a family. Even if the job isn't complete by the end of the fifteen minutes, something about feeling like they are all on my side lightens my mental load.

I don't really care if he doesn't feel the same way about the mess that I do or if he doesn't know where something is kept on occasion. What I do care about is whether he rallies when I need him to. And he almost always does.

The honest truth is that the partner who isn't bothered by the mental load is probably more mentally healthy. Or at least a little more chill. It wouldn't hurt us as moms to let go a little more and not worry so much about the messes and the chaos that motherhood brings to our lives.

The Most Important Part Is That We're a Team When It Matters

The takeaway is this: yes, historically women feel the mental load a lot more than men. But that's OK. You can both work hard at shifting in your marriage.

After all, if same-sex couples can share the mental load more evenly, why can't heterosexual couples?

So now that we know it is possible to share the mental load a little more evenly, how exactly do we do it?

Constant communication is key.
You have to talk about the mental load to share it. Your spouse may seem like he sleeps a little too soundly at night, making you believe his mental load is nonexistent. But on the flip side, he probably has no idea how many tabs you have open in your brain unless you verbalize it. You have to understand that you could be married to someone who isn't bothered by the same things you're bothered by. But talking it through can save you both a lot of mental anguish

and bitterness that the other person isn't doing their part. The key to fixing it all is to talk about the mental load. In the beginning it might be every single day until you're both in the habit of sharing all there is to do.

Talk about your worries with your partner.
Tell him everything you're worried about. If he finds it helpful, you can even make a written list, and he can pick things off that list throughout the week to lighten your mental load.

Return the favor when your partner gets overwhelmed. It's all about teamwork.
If you see your partner feeling stressed, check in and ask what you can do to help. His list will not look like your list, but if you recognize he also has a mental load, just checking in with him might be enough to make his mental load lighter.

Mental Load and Marriage

Like every wife throughout history, I could write a book on how much I love my husband and how crazy he makes me.

On the other hand, I wouldn't even be able to count how many times I have questioned internally and out loud why he married me.

We are complete opposites in so many ways.

I always joke that the first time I went to eat at his family's house for dinner, it felt like something out of the movie *My Big Fat Greek Wedding*.

It was just his parents, us, and his great aunt. Everyone was very proper, saying things like "please" and "thank you" as they passed around the potatoes. There were no outbursts of laughter or arguing. There were no interruptions and no cross words.

I remember almost getting panicky inside. *What is this?* I wondered. And then it hit me—everyone was just so *polite*.

It was a completely foreign experience to me. I felt like the girl in *My Big Fat Greek Wedding* who was holding on to this big secret that my family was nothing like this one.

In fact, because I had gone away to college in my husband's home state, I spent a lot of time with his family when we were dating, but the reverse was not true. And a small part of me was relieved. I was worried I would scare away this great guy I really liked who obviously came from the most polite family on the planet.

What would he think of my family's inappropriate conversations at the dinner table? My grandma was notorious for bringing up something 100 percent disgusting and inappropriate every time we gathered with her for dinner. It almost always centered around bowel movements or the lack thereof.

My family talks loudly over each other, and while we are Southern and have basic human decency built into us, we aren't exactly what I would call polite. We speak our minds, and we are sarcastic and loud. We often told jokes at dinner, and a fight breaking out would not be out of the norm for us.

Unlike my husband's family, mine was as crazy as they came. While I knew nothing different growing up, when I sat down to dinner with my husband's family, the truth became obvious very quickly.

While my husband grew up mountain biking, skiing, and rock climbing, I grew up fishing, playing outside with friends, and spending too much time on video games.

He loves to be active, and I love to stay home.

The differences between our likes and dislikes are too numerous to name. Even twenty years into marriage, my husband and I are still baffled by how two people so different could end up falling in love. We are the epitome of how opposites attract.

When we were young and naïve, it seemed exciting to experience new things together that the other had not. I tried hard to be adventurous with him, and he tried to watch movies with me even though it was hard for him to sit still.

Compromise Is Easy When You're Young and in Love

It was easier to make those compromises because we were young. The only compromises we had to make were with each other. Instead of navigating the fickle moods of an entire household, we just had to figure out how to live with and love each other. Although it wasn't perfect in those pre-kid days, it was a challenging reality I could manage.

So although it was never perfect, we didn't have nearly the road bumps we've had since kids have come along.

Then, almost exactly four years into our marriage, we were suddenly a family of three. Two and a half years after that, and bam! We were a family of four. When we became a family of five, it seemed to push us both to our limits.

It wasn't long after kids came along that my anxiety was affecting my marriage.

The mental load and my mental health issues are not to blame for my marriage struggles. They are simply one factor out of many. Both of us forgot that we were really important to each other for a few years.

Recently, my husband and I had a big blow-up. I said some awful, regrettable things. I threw the D word out there. I told him I wanted him to leave. And I felt an anger that I could not stop as I hurled hurtful words out at him. They just kept coming.

I told him later that it felt like an out-of-body experience. I could not control the dark thoughts that were coming into my head:

He doesn't love me.
This is hopeless.
I can't go on.
This marriage is over.
I'm not lovable.

But worse, I couldn't control the words coming out of my mouth in rapid succession aimed directly at him. Face-to-face I screamed—yes, screamed (thank goodness our children were asleep)—awful, terrible things.

He was quiet as I went on my rageful tirade.

When I was finished, he responded with something like, "That really hurt" and left the room.

I was stunned, and in an instant, I was so ashamed.

I knew at that moment that what I did next would affect what happened to us. We had been in therapy for a few months, and we were both trying to fix things, but we obviously had so much to work on still.

I knew that I had to go to him. I felt so much horror at what I had said that I felt embarrassed. But I knew I had to go to him because I was more afraid than embarrassed.

It took courage to apologize. When I walked into the room, I stood next to him as he sat looking at something on the computer. I found out later in therapy that he was looking for a hotel room to stay in that night. I sobbed and covered my face and said, "I'm so sorry. I didn't mean it. I didn't mean it."

He got up and hugged me as I fell into his arms.

Uncontrollable sobs overcame my body in that moment. I apologized and told him that I didn't want him to leave. I needed him. I told him that I was not in control and that I was depressed and scared.

It was a pivotal moment in our relationship. By being extremely vulnerable with him at that moment, I believe that I changed the trajectory of our relationship by admitting my own defeat.

I knew the root of this fight was because my brain was telling me lies. I was tired, angry, and depressed and had been for over a year. After three kids and almost twenty years of marriage, I was utterly exhausted.

But on top of that, I was not practicing self-care and I was not on the right medication. Our kids were getting older, and the mental load I carried by trying to have it all was too much.

I had to wave the white flag to save our marriage. I had to be vulnerable and admit defeat. I had to make more of an effort. Some things had to go on the back burner while we got our collective stuff figured out.

Looking back, I can see things I did that were detrimental, and I know it was because my mental load was heavy and my mental health was suffering. My mom brain was one big hot, sweaty mess.

The Mental Load Isn't Meant to Be Carried Alone

A smart therapist (Esther Perel, LMFT) once said, "Most people are going to have two or three marriages or committed relationships in their adult life. Some of us will have them with the same person."

We have to talk to our partners about the mental load we carry, or it will hurt us in the long run. So what does that look like?

Be authentic.
Taking the steps to be our true authentic selves has to start with showing the people we love most who we are. Vulnerability is showing up to our partners as who we are in each moment, even if who we are is never exactly the same. We will inevitably change throughout our marriages,

but we have to share those changes with the person with whom we chose to share our lives.

Be vulnerable.

Being vulnerable and saying we can't do something and we need help will release us from pain and make our burdens seem lighter. Brené Brown says, "Vulnerability is not winning or losing; it's having the courage to show up and be seen when we have no control over the outcome. Vulnerability is not weakness; it's our greatest measure of courage."

Letting someone else understand the depth and scope of your burden will help you feel like you have someone willing to throw you a life raft when you desperately need it. It is courageous to ask for help to lighten your mental load.

When I waved the proverbial white flag during the fight with my husband, he reached for me and held me. And while we still have our struggles and arguments, my vulnerability that night brought us together instead of tearing us apart.

Honesty and vulnerability go hand in hand. It takes bravery to tell your truth, even when you've been married a long time. It isn't always pretty to peek inside your brain. But

> Brené Brown says, "Vulnerability is not winning or losing; it's having the courage to show up and be seen when we have no control over the outcome. Vulnerability is not weakness; it's our greatest measure of courage."

by being honest, we show that we trust our partner with even our deepest hurts.

Don't make it a competition.

I recently saw on Facebook a chart made by a wife where she had all her mental load tally items tacked to a wall. Two things were obvious: she hadn't been married that long, and there were no kids involved yet. She said it created a major shift in her marriage for her husband to have a visual of who was doing what in their marriage.

I cringed a little. I try not to judge what other people do, but I guarantee you that my husband would see that little chart as a threat. It's tempting to tally, like she was doing, in chart form, but in some relationships that could be damaging.

Have a sincere conversation first, and if your husband wants a chart to mark off, great. Communication is key. Don't keep throwing it in his face that you do more. That will never help.

Seek professional help.

Marriage therapy saved our marriage, and I tell that to everyone that I can. Every couple should seek therapy. You are worth it. Your marriage is worth it.

Marriages are about bringing together two wildly different people and making a new life together. And more often than not we just don't have the skills or emotional capacity to figure that out on our own.

CHAPTER 3

The Need to Be Seen

Have you heard people say, "The Lord doesn't give you more than you can handle"? I believe that. But on some days I want to scream, "Really, Lord? I *know* I can't handle this."

In fact, I may have said those very words out loud a few times. But in the end, I do handle it. And usually, I've learned a lesson in the process.

An outsider might look at my life and see a great husband with a good job, a cute house, and three beautiful kids. It would be easy to think that I have a cushy life.

Or that I don't appreciate what I have. The truth is, I have my struggles too—they're just, often, completely concealed from the world around me.

The mental load of motherhood is exactly that: a struggle in our mind that is tailor-made for us. It's exhausting and overwhelming, and every single one of us has some struggle going on while we fumble our way through motherhood.

I remember sitting at a dinner once with some family, and they were discussing cancer that a family member had recently gone through. There was a lot of back-and-forth about how strong and resilient the person was for fighting through something was so hard.

I didn't disagree. I watched this family member battle with something extremely difficult. Cancer had robbed her of so much. I admired her positivity through it all. I rarely (if at all) heard her utter a word of complaint.

But what I will never forget is when she turned to me and acknowledged that I have had struggles with my anxiety.

I was stunned, frankly, and grateful that one person saw what I was going through. Because when you live with a hidden illness, it's easy to hide it. But it's also easy to feel incredibly alone and that no one gets it.

The need to be seen, I believe, is a vital part of dealing with the mental pressures of motherhood. If only someone understood us. If only someone would acknowledge us in our suffering. If only someone could say, "Me too" when it came to whatever we are struggling with.

I believe that's why there are so many forums, online groups, TikToks, and Instagram accounts out there trying to bring women together in this unique experience of motherhood. We want to be seen.

Yet at the same time, few people in our worlds know the real us. We have this deep inner conflict to keep our real problems hidden from everyone, and simultaneously we want to be seen! It makes zero sense whatsoever.

The intense need by every human to be seen and understood is what connects us to each other. Women raising babies need this.

On a girls' trip recently I woke up around 2:00 a.m. with extreme nausea. At first, I thought I had eaten something bad at dinner. I was in the bathroom waiting for the inevitable. I became so overwhelmed, I lay down on the cold, disgusting hotel bathroom floor, and suddenly I realized I wasn't sick at all; I was having a panic attack.

Two of my best friends were just on the other side of the wall. I thought about calling out to them, but I was in a vulnerable position. Instead, I laid on that bathroom floor for two hours crying and trying to hold it together.

When the anxiety subsided, I got up and crawled back into bed, and my friends were none the wiser.

Why? Was it because I didn't want to be seen crying? Or was it because I didn't want to interrupt their sleep?

The next morning, I told them what had happened, and they were incredibly pissed at me. These were my best friends, and I didn't reach out.

While it was embarrassing being on the bathroom floor crying about my problems at 2:00 a.m. in a hotel room, it was more embarrassing to tell them about it after the fact.

If I had allowed them to see me being vulnerable, I guarantee we would have grown even closer as a result. What a gift that would be to all of us.

What Does Being Seen Actually Do for Us?

Previously, I discussed how my husband and I went through a rocky time in our marriage. To be honest, marriage therapy saved it. We still go, although not nearly as often, just to have time to reconnect.

But when I really stop to think about it, marriage therapy for us has been mostly a way for us to truly see each other. It was in that small office on that leather couch where my anger and bitterness melted, and I saw my husband for who he really is at his core.

I saw the person I married. I also saw the person he was after three kids and twenty years of marriage. I loved both parts of him. We had both changed, but seeing each other made us feel closer.

The beauty in all those tear-filled sessions was that I felt seen too. He saw my heart when I could talk about things with vulnerability and not so much heightened emotion. You know, the kind of emotions you feel when exhausted and irrational, your hair is in a hysterical messy bun, and you feel like a swamp rat. You are trying to cook dinner after dealing with the kids all day, and he has a salty comment about the soup. Well, the last thing I want to hear is that the soup is too salty. He almost ended up wearing the salty soup!

My husband gets me at my worst in those moments, and my emotional side almost always takes over. I'm tired. I'm stressed, and he can keep his salty comments to himself.

Marriage therapy helped us see each other again through intentional conversations. We also realized that we wanted and needed validation.

Validation is what we're all really looking for.

According to Dr. Kristalyn Salters-Pedneault, when people validate our emotions, they accept us for who we are, and we sense that we are important to them. As a result, we feel more connected. Some research has shown that emotional validation may even help us better regulate our emotions.[3]

One study[4] revealed that mothers used social media to seek validation about mothering. There was a positive correlation between women who posted photos about their babies and how they felt about their own mothering.

I found that fascinating. It shows that finding people who see us and what we are going through will help us see ourselves better too.

In my many hours of writing online and sharing my own struggles, I've realized that we each have hurdles that affect our own mental load about mothering.

I know people who struggle with financial issues or have a child with a disability. Some families struggle with loss or infertility. Others with divorce or abuse. Still others deal with drug addiction and extended family turmoil.

Those are just the things we can see on the outside. But some mothers struggle with things that simply can't be seen.

While one person might sail through their child's food allergies and consider it no big deal, another might be crippled by it. We are all unique.

We all handle things differently.

I sat with a friend one night at dinner a couple of years ago as she shared some struggles.

As I listened to her talk about a trial with one of her kids, I was amazed. I was amazed at her strength. Amazed at her commitment to motherhood. Amazed at the things she was willing to do to fight and advocate for her child. I was thinking, *I don't know if I could fight that battle like she is every day. She is such a good mom.*

Most people wouldn't even know she's going through a major battle just looking at her. She's so well put together—hair done, eyelash extensions, and a cute outfit seemingly right out of a magazine. People who pass her in the grocery store probably don't know the sleepless nights she's had or the constant battles she's been fighting in her own home.

Mothers fight battles every day that no one sees. It's a beautiful thing if you stop to think about it, because we get the rare opportunity to raise the children whom we've been given and help them overcome life's hurdles.

So to the mother who's fighting her own battle right now, I see you.

I see your struggles to keep it together when the toddler is giving you his fifteenth battle of wills for the day.

I see you, mama, fighting at IEP meetings for your special needs child, wading through mounds of paperwork that moms with neurotypical children would never dream of having to do simply to enroll their kids in school.

I am talking to you, the mom with mental illness. The one who takes a pill every day to be there for her kids. To be strong. To fight. And to be the mom that she never had.

I ache for you mamas fighting battles of chronic illness. You suffer through physical pain while doing a physically demanding job day in and day out.

I see the mom who tries so hard and feels like she's failing because she's a perfectionist and wants to get it just right. The battle she fights is with herself. To keep up. To constantly be doing better than she did the day before. To control her environment so she can feel safe.

I see moms who fight to be both parents for their kids and have the heartache of explaining why the other half isn't there. They suffer in silence when their child asks about the other parent and they have no answers. They struggle to put a meal on the table, and no one even knows about it.

To the moms who fight a defiant child, or just a strong-willed one, you battle every day to find the balance between giving in to the child with a strong personality whom you love fiercely, and teaching her that no, she can't have everything she wants and won't always get her way. I see that you're most likely raising a future leader who will make big changes one day.

Mothers fight battles every day that no one sees.

I see you, the mom who battles every day trying to balance it all. Be it all. Have it all.

I see the mom who battles for self-control with her weight and the one who battles to give self-esteem to her own kids when she doesn't feel like she has any of her own.

There are moms who struggle not to give up on the kid whom the world has already given up on. Who are willing to take on the brave role of foster mom or adopt a child who is longing to be wanted.

Some moms have empty arms. They haven't gotten to hold their babies for longer than a few hours, days, or weeks.

We all fight our battles. Often in silence. Sometimes alone. But we fight them anyway.

Maybe you're fighting one right now. One that you don't dare share with even a close friend for fear of breaking down or being judged. Or worse, for feeling like a bad mother because you complain a little about how hard your battle is.

While we may not feel like we're making a lick of headway in our battles, the fact that we haven't thrown in the towel means we're stronger than we realized. Heck, we got out of bed this morning. (That has to count for something!) We didn't even leave that middle child to hitchhike his way home this afternoon as we threatened. Instead, we chose to show up and fight for our kids, our marriage, and our mental health.

That's what moms do. We fight. We advocate. We don't give up. We battle within ourselves and outside ourselves. We are willing to do the hard stuff that breaks our hearts into millions of pieces.

Because we know all the quiet (and not-so-quiet) battles in the world are worth it. Because motherhood is worth it. Every last bit.

How Can We See and Validate the Invisible Battles?

Consider these ideas:

Give grace to other women.
We can't see each other's struggles, so let's give other women

around us more grace. Forgive our friends more often when they don't text back. Let it go when they say something you know they don't mean. Support them in their battles.

Listen more intently.
Behind every mother's struggle are hints that it's there. If we listen more closely, we will be able to ask questions to help our friends open up. Show empathy when they share something you don't understand. Tell them you are there for them. Show up without being asked. Work on validating them despite not going through the same thing.

Be more open with your own struggles.
When we are more vulnerable and share our trials, it gives others permission to do the same. Share your hurt and pain with those you trust, and they will in turn feel safe to share their hurt.

We don't have to experience the same trial to be able to validate and see the struggles of someone else. Whether it's your spouse or a friend, we can simply be a safe space for others to be seen. And we might find lifelong friends and loyal partners in the process.

CHAPTER 4

But I Love My Children!

When you're parenting, you're in a constant tug-of-war with not only your own feelings, emotions, and mental well-being, but also those of your children.

It's impossible to balance it all every day perfectly. Many mothers like myself feel so incredibly overwhelmed by new motherhood that it's all-consuming.

Motherhood is a constant balancing act of trying to determine what needs to be prioritized. You feel like you're a ringmaster at a circus.

Someone spills the popcorn and starts crying.

The tigers are let loose.

The tent catches fire.

Then out jump the creepy clowns.

It's funny to think about motherhood that way, but when you're the one expected to keep all the balls in the air,

> Motherhood is a constant balancing act of trying to determine what needs to be prioritized. You feel like you're a ringmaster at a circus.

all while you're losing your own balance on the tightrope, it can lead any mom to depression and anxiety.

As mothers, we are naturally predisposed to feel responsible for all the circus chaos.

What's the result on our mental health if we feel this gigantic weight that no one else seems to feel?

It begs the question: why do we do this to ourselves?

Why Does Anyone Want to Become a Mother?

I had fears early on that I wasn't meant to be a mother. And now sixteen years into motherhood I don't think it matters anymore whether I was meant to be one. I made that choice; I'm a mom to three beautiful humans. This is my circus and my monkeys. And I love my kids. Promise.

I have zero regrets about becoming a mother, but insecurities often cloud our view of the experience. We feel afraid to talk about the hard parts of parenting because someone is always there to tell us we aren't grateful enough.

Every mother knows that the rewards that come from motherhood are worth it. But we always hear women qualify their complaints with the obligatory, "But I love my children! I really do!"

Of *course* we do. Why do we always add this to the end of every sentence when we're saying it's hard?

I look back at my time as a new mother, and in some ways, it traumatized me. I know that sounds dramatic, but when I was in it, I felt so overwhelmed and insecure that I do think trauma was involved.

We don't talk about how early motherhood isn't always bonding and butterflies. Early motherhood is crying when your baby is crying and sleep deprivation and extreme fear.

It was most likely my own trauma from childhood bubbling up in a way I've still yet to fully understand as a mom, but I do think that being a mom was hard for me in the beginning. I struggled with postpartum depression and postpartum anxiety with every baby.

I felt like I was an emotional mess, barely keeping my head above water. Some days I was a complete disaster. There were days when I questioned not just my abilities but also my life choices. And my biggest fear of all was that I wasn't enjoying it enough.

You can't possibly enjoy every second.

It's always annoyed me that I felt this immense pressure to soak it all in and "enjoy every second." I hated that phrase. I still do. If I listen to my body, it creates a physical response in my gut when I hear, "Enjoy every second; it goes so fast!"

I know it's well-intentioned, and I totally understand the sentiment better now that the empty nest years are closer than those little kid years. But I was a terrified new mom. I lived in constant fear of so many things.

I was afraid I was screwing it up.

I was afraid they would die.

I was afraid I yelled too much or didn't have enough patience. Patience is a hard one.

I was afraid when they would cry a little too long or cough in the night.

I was afraid my anxiety would be my undoing.

I was afraid I was traumatizing them in some way.

I was afraid if they missed a nap or got a fever.

I was afraid that they were too messy, or fought too much, or were too emotional, or not emotional enough.

I was afraid of germs.

I was afraid that my husband didn't love me the same way anymore.

Lord, have mercy; I was afraid of all of it.

And because I lived in a perpetual state of fear back then, I was also afraid I was missing the good stuff because the bad stuff felt so overwhelming.

I have trauma around some very real things that seem almost silly to me now. But I don't wish to minimize how they felt in the moment.

One particularly bad winter when our (then) two children were about five and one, we were in limbo between houses. We were waiting for our house out of state to sell and had moved in with my recently widowed father-in-law. We had overtaken his house with our little family, so he moved into the guest room (bless his generous heart), and my husband and I took the master.

The master bedroom was gigantic and had this huge walk-in closet. It was so big, in fact, that the closet became our youngest's bedroom. I kid you not, our son slept in a closet for almost eight months. It's fine. Totally fine.

I spent my days trying to get acclimated to a new state, make friends at story time, and count down the seconds until my husband got home from his new job so he could help out with our babies.

Then, we decided an outing to the mall would be fun so the kids could spend some energy before bed.

This mall had a train that would take the kids around the loop of the storefronts, and my sweet husband told me to go shopping alone while he took the kids on the train.

I was thrilled to have some alone time, even though I knew it would be short. I just didn't know how short.

About ten minutes into my kid-free bliss, my phone rang. It was my husband.

"I need you to meet me in front of Claire's."

"What's wrong?" I said in my innocent I-didn't-know-what-was-coming way.

"She just threw up everywhere. All over me. All over the train. They had to get a roll of paper towels. It wasn't enough. I just had to leave them cleaning up all the mess because it's all over us. We need to leave. Now."

I don't remember much that happened after that. We somehow got home with a vomit-covered child who smelled like chicken nuggets and parmesan cheese. But the worst was still to come.

Within a few minutes of getting her home, bathed, and settled, the baby started projectile vomiting.

Thankfully, my father-in-law had two bathrooms, both of which we were about to put to good use. I don't know

now how we got through that night, but I have this vivid memory of one specific moment.

My husband and I passed each other around 2:00 a.m. in the big open hallway that divided one side of the house from the other. He was taking one kid's vomit-soaked clothes to the laundry, and I was getting up to deal with a vomiting baby who needed a bath.

It's almost a tender memory now, both of us working together to take care of this little family we built together before we knew there would be so much puke involved. But at the time, it felt like too much for my weary soul. Was this it?

Is this the part that I'm supposed to be enjoying? Hell, no. No, thank you. This *sucks*.

I didn't sign up for puke fests at 2:00 a.m. by two children who can only aim their projectile chicken nuggies everywhere that is not a toilet.

There is a big chunk of the new motherhood years that sucks the life out of you. You catch vomit in your hands. You wipe the sweat from your brow only to accidentally smear poop in its place. You walk around in circles with a tiny human who is inconsolable in the wee hours of the night, and you question how you'll ever make it to the years when they finally puke in the toilet and sulk in their rooms trying to get away from you.

The pukefest of 2010 still haunts me. I'm not going to lie. It overshadows some of the good stuff. I can laugh at it now, but I wonder if I missed the good stuff because that bad stuff was *really* bad. My anxiety at the time made it even worse.

Don't worry; we do enjoy enough of it.

Recently, sixteen years into being a mom, an old home video popped up in my Facebook memories. My middle kid loves to watch these with me and frequently grabs my phone and laughs at things I wrote about them in their baby and toddler years. One day we were watching a video, and I was mesmerized—as I always am now—at what was happening in our little world when my kids were babies.

I had forgotten so much of it.

My youngest couldn't walk yet and was in his footed, zip-up jammies, and my middle was next to me on the couch giggling as he tried out my back scratcher inside his favorite pajamas.

They looked fresh out of the bath, and the baby was whining. It was background noise to me at the time. He was my third, and my focus was always split between three kids six and under.

As my now thirteen-year-old and I watched the video, we laughed at the way he said certain words. The whole video was full of smiles and giggles.

I wasn't completely visible in the video frame, but I can picture her—me. I can picture the mom I was back then.

I could hear in my voice that I was tired. My hair was probably in a messy bun at the end of a long day. A part of me was probably waiting for the clock to hit that magical time when I could put the kids in bed and have some rare alone time with my husband or pass out in front of a TV show.

The furniture in the video is long gone now, as are the old box TV and the mismatched thrifted couch and orange vintage chair. None of that is important, but it's weird to take a step back into another time with a fresh perspective. We were younger. Poorer. And inexperienced.

I could hear my voice in the video. Calm and patient. Laughing. Pointing out things to my middle. Engaging with the baby. Tickling their bellies.

As we watched the video together, a thought came over me that whispered to my heart: *See? You* did *enjoy it.*

And mamas, I did.

I watched that video with the eyes of a veteran mother who still struggles but no longer feels totally incapable, inadequate, and riddled with guilt.

I watched it with the eyes of someone new. I'm not the same woman I was ten or so years ago. Far from it, in fact. I am not afraid like I once was. Sure, I have worries still— every mother does. But I'm not afraid of some of the things that crippled me as a new mom.

Motherhood Wrecked Me in the Beginning

I would argue that new motherhood, with the weight of those lives in my hands, traumatized me a little. It was a lot of responsibility and pressure.

It was also a lot of poop, pee, puke, and tears.

Although it still is a lot of responsibility and pressure, the physical demands are subsiding. I have two teenagers now, and my youngest thinks he's running this place most days. I'm in a different stage of life than I was all those years ago. I'm guilty of feeling what those other moms have always told me: it does go so fast.

But I feel comforted by the fact that I enjoyed it, y'all. I saw it in that video. I look back and recognize that I had a lot of moments like that too. That video of me soaking it all in was not the only one. I spent a lot of time just watching my kids grow. Videotaping them. Taking pictures. Soaking it up. And those memories float back into my life now via old Facebook videos and photos, and guess what? I get to enjoy it again through their teenage eyes with them.

It seems like the empty nest moms are always trying to tell us that it goes so fast. It goes so fast, yes, but—and this is *super* important—the fact that it goes so fast is not the point. The point is, if you're feeling inadequate and scared and overwhelmed at the weight of motherhood—the mental load you carry—and you're feeling the pressure of not enjoying it enough, just know that it's OK. We were never meant to enjoy all of it.

Even I, who has many years of parenting under her belt, am guilty of telling a mom friend that it goes so fast. At the time, she had two little ones, ages four and two, and we were staying with them as we did a lot of sightseeing. With children underfoot, it took so long for us to get anywhere, which instantly catapulted me back to that stage of life— when just getting out of the house is an ordeal.

One kid didn't want to wear a pink shirt because it was too scratchy; the other one couldn't find his matching shoes. We didn't have the right sippy cup, and there was a bug to be inspected in great detail on the windowsill.

Feeding them was an ordeal. Bananas that had histori- cally been an acceptable fruit option were suddenly inedible. The cereal was too crunchy. The toast was too toasty.

Switching and installing car seats in our car rental was an ordeal. Enough said.

Missed naps were OK some days and devastating other days. On the worst days, the missed naps caused the whole afternoon activity to go off the rails. Nothing was good or right in the world. Kids flattened themselves in parking lots not wanting to walk anymore. Toddlers acted drunk. It was total chaos.

I had that wide-eyed emoji look the whole time we were together. Because I had forgotten so much of what it took to just keep a child that age alive, fed, and clean, let alone happy and emotionally stable.

Yikes, it was exhausting, and I was right back in the thick of it with her, but also I was kind of like, *Oh my gosh, I'm so glad I'm past that stage.*

No, I did not say that to her.

I said something worse, though. I said, "It's true what they say: it goes by so fast." I hope I didn't say to enjoy it too; honestly, I can't remember if I did or not.

I immediately wanted to punch myself in the face. I swear I had vowed not to be that person. I was not going to be that annoying mom who would ever say that to a mom, and yet it flowed out of my mouth before I could even stop it, and I felt like I was having an out-of-body experience.

I immediately stammered, "Oh my gosh, I'm so sorry I said that. I swore I would never say that." My husband laughed at me because he knew how much I hated that phrase. I chastised myself inwardly and felt like a hypocrite. Who had I become? I just wanted to reassure her (with the best intentions) it would get better, but instead, I placed a burden on her already overwhelmed heart.

While I have now found that statement to be true as I look back, it is still not something moms want to hear when they are in the trenches of young motherhood.

My story is an example of how even those of us nearly wrecked by motherhood can quickly forget how hard it was in the beginning. But I think it's OK that we forget some of the hard stuff. It's proof that we aren't supposed to enjoy every single second anyway.

New Motherhood Comes at a Cost

Your sleep-deprived body isn't going to possibly have the capacity to soak up every moment. Some things are lost. That's just the way it is designed. Your vomit-soaked clothes are never going to smell nice in the moment (or ever, let's be honest). The colicky baby won't bring you joy when he's arching his back and refusing to be put down or held.

We can accept that new motherhood can suck royally, and we don't have to add the caveat, "But I love my children! I promise."

It may not feel like it when you're in the middle of it, but you're doing the best you can. You may not be enjoying all of it, but you're enjoying enough.

You're taking the pictures and breathing in their clean heads after a bath, and you're watching them closely as they toddle around.

You're amazed at the things they learn despite your inadequacies, and you're feeling those chubby toddler arms around your neck. You tickle bellies and teach them about the world, and you read one more story when you can.

I promise you: in the moment you may not feel good enough or strong enough or even sane enough. But you are doing it. Every day. Even when your bones are tired and your soul is sucked dry. You're doing it.

You're enjoying it too. Just the right amount.

CHAPTER 5

Showers Are a Necessity . . . Not Self Care

As a mom to three kids, I've heard it more than once: *put yourself first, and you'll be a better mom.* It's true, and I know it, but the idea of self-care gets confusing when you are depressed, anxious, overwhelmed, and so on.

It seems the idea of self-care is a popular one. You can browse Pinterest or any website or magazine that targets women, and I guarantee you will find an article on the importance of self-care.

Taking time for yourself and making yourself a priority is always being marketed to women.

It took me a long time as a new mom to realize what self-care was and what it wasn't. I remember when my son's fifth birthday party was coming up. I decided I wanted something easy because it was the dead of winter, but I was struggling to come up with easy ideas.

Then I ran across a pancakes and pajamas–themed party. *Perfect.* I could invite the boys over for pancakes, in their pajamas, and then we would have a dance party in the basement.

Done.

Somewhere in the middle of enjoying my newfound idea of an "easy" birthday party, I lost my sanity.

I decided I needed to decorate. Because five-year-old boys clearly care about decorations. I swear to you, I must have been browsing Pinterest, seen varying degrees of this "easy" birthday party, and lost my marbles. Now I know not to trust anything on Pinterest that claims it is easy or stress-free. *And* how the only true thirty-minute dinner recipe is to order pizza.

I imagined each child getting a perfectly groomed stack of pancakes on a picture-perfect plate with cute toothpick flags stuck in their stack. Why flags? I don't know.

I began to take cute and colorful washi tape rolls from my crafting supplies and make flags for stacks of pancakes. Some were red and white striped, some blue, green plaid, red with stars.

This was going to be the cutest stack of pancakes that ever existed in the "momosphere."

I even enlisted my seven-year-old to help make them. But tiny miniature pancake flags didn't seem like enough without some pom-poms. I was going to thread, string, and hang colorful pom-poms for decoration. Store-bought Paw Patrol decorations are for moms who don't love their children. I made a cute banner that I spent too much time on.

This party had to be Pinterest-worthy and *handmade*.

When the night before the party rolled around, there I was: an extremely busy mom with three kids under seven years old. And unfinished pom-pom décor.

I had a choice to make. I could either stay up until 2:00 a.m. stabbing myself in the fingers to thread little poofs into a garland before hosting breakfast for a crowd of wild, sweaty boys, or I could take care of me. And put *me* to bed early.

I left the pom-poms sitting there. Unopened.

The kids came at 9:00 a.m., we ate pancakes, and I don't even remember if I used the washi tape toothpick flags. I don't recall the boys gushing over their care and craftsmanship, and I also don't have any pained memories of them, ripe with indignation, refusing to eat their pancakes until they were properly adorned. It's almost like five-year-olds don't care about Pinterest-perfect parties (they really don't) and we just enjoy driving ourselves crazy for no good reason.

What I do remember is the boys had a blast. I'm more likely to remember that because I was well-rested enough to deal with their shenanigans.

It taught me a powerful lesson about self-care and motherhood: not being the best at everything you do can be the absolute best form of self-care. I know you have heard that whole thing about not being able to pour from an empty cup. It's true.

Your kids are not going to care about pom-pom banners anyway. They really don't care.

What the World Doesn't Tell Us About Self-Care

As a young mom, I used to think that self-care meant pedicures, dinner with a friend, and a girls' night out dancing at the club. (That makes me laugh.) Now, with age, wisdom, and knees that sound like microwave popcorn, I can confidently say I would rather bathe with knives while listening to a Pokémon TED Talk than spend a night out dancing at any club or bar.

Self-care sounds awesome, but it's not realistic to find that much time for myself. Yet that is what we're told to do to find some relief from the demands of motherhood.

Sometimes self-care does not look like going out with friends. Self-care just looks like chilling out when it comes to pom-pom décor and little, tiny flags.

> **Not being the best at everything you do can be the absolute best form of self-care.**

When you're depressed, self-care can be lying in bed all day. And that's OK.

The reality is that self-care the way we see it on TV, like spa treatments and mimosas at brunch, can feel overwhelming and time-consuming.

Allowing yourself your own feelings is the ultimate form of self-care. Tell yourself that it's OK if you are doing x, y, and z because you are feeling empty, lonely, anxious, afraid, burnt out . . . sound familiar?

And for most moms, our days are full. We are running around with brains overflowing with to-do lists, and the thought of self-care can sound downright exhausting.

Karaoke with friends at 9:00 p.m. when my bed is so inviting and warm and does not have children in it? No, thanks. I have an important thing I need to do, like watch Netflix and fall asleep at 9:00 p.m.

Going out with friends, or to the spa, or to a family gathering is the last thing you need when you are feeling low or anxious. Often what you need is space.

Space to slow down. Space to slow your brain and your body.

While I firmly believe self-care can make us better mothers, the world doesn't make self-care sound simple. Giving ourselves space in this universe (both figuratively and literally) from responsibilities and children can work miracles in the mind of someone who is mentally overwhelmed.

I'm a big fan of self-care. Five out of five stars. In fact, it took me years and a little bit (OK—a lot) of therapy to realize that self-care is essential to our emotional well-being as mothers. No one can give what they don't have energy or capacity to share.

When I was a new mom, my self-care was nonexistent. I was a nursing machine, consumed with this new squirmy, squishy being who needed my constant attention. I was convinced my husband could do nothing right.

Yes. I was one of *those* new moms. I rarely let that new baby out of my sight, even when her perfectly capable father was around to do things.

I hovered and flitted around like a gnat to watch how he changed the diaper and how he held her and how he did literally everything.

It wasn't until I matured, had a couple more kids under my roof, and realized my husband was not only capable but was the father of *our* children that I realized the kids were his responsibility as well. Then I started to explore what I needed as a person to feel whole.

Self-Care Is Crucial to Our Survival

What the world often doesn't say is that self-care isn't just important, it's crucial to our survival as moms.

With depression and anxiety in my DNA, I had to learn how to balance new motherhood with my mental illness. A key factor in finding that balance was realizing I wasn't just pouring from an empty cup, I was pouring from an empty cup in the Sahara Desert. There was no water in sight, and I was drowning.

It turns out that without self-care, I became angry and resentful, not to mention depressed and anxious, lashing out at everyone around me. In short, without self-care, I was a shell of a human being.

Fast forward a few years, and I've learned to ask for what I need. I've learned that I need more time away from my children than I thought.

I need quiet hours (yes, hours) alone to revive my introverted little heart and soul.

There is a message popping up on pretty Instagram accounts and in Facebook mom groups about self-care that can be misleading and downright damaging.

The message? That basic human needs are self-care.

As women, our load is so great that we expect that taking any time for ourselves is the equivalent of self-care.

We have seen the funny memes and captions lamenting how long our husbands spend in the bathroom doing their business, and yet a mom will post that her time in the bathroom is a mini vacation from her kids. Is it?

Or how about the message we see from a mom on our Instagram feed that she is taking a trip alone to Target as her self-care?

I'm sorry, but a trip alone to Target is nice (and sometimes quite enjoyable), but for me, it's also usually filled with my mental checklist of things my family needs.

My husband is out of deodorant.

My daughter needs new socks—no-show ones. Didn't she ask for white?

Do we have eggs at home for dinner later? Are we out of dog food?

It's fine if you really love going to Target alone and that is your form of self-care. However, I would suggest carefully asking yourself if this is restorative self-care, because honestly, when I go to Target alone, it's still filled with texts like, "When are you going to be home, Mom?" and, "Do you know where my soccer cleats are?"

I don't know about you, but that doesn't feel

rejuvenating while I browse the dollar bins for more pump-kin décor I don't need.

Self-care absolutely can look different for everyone. But be careful not to tout basic human needs as self-care. Basic needs such as the following:

- *Eating a meal* or having a cup of hot coffee should not be a form of self-care. It is basic human care. I mean, coffee is a must-have for some.
- *Taking a hot shower* is warm and inviting, and it's fun how you can hear your own thoughts for a min-ute between the phantom baby cries while the baby is asleep, but again, this is a basic human need.
- *Going to the bathroom* alone with the door locked is not self-care (unless you're taking a thirty-minute poop scrolling your phone and avoiding the family, like husbands are infamous for).
- *Chasing a toddler* at the park is not exercise you can call self-care. It's literally preventing a child from dying as they catapult their body off the top of the monkey bars because they think they can fly.
- *Taking a sick day* when you're sick is not self-care. It's a sick day. One you deserve. Hopefully it's not accompanied by a sick kid or two as well.
- *Going to the doctor* for a routine visit is something you need to do to stay well. This is not self-care.

I could go on, but these are some of the many things that I hear women say they are doing for self-care.

Frankly, self-care needs a little more thought and effort put into it than folding laundry with AirPods in your ears while listening to a book on tape.

That's multitasking more than self-care.

The good news is that you get to decide what self-care looks like to you.

Self-care is something that we do on purpose to take care of ourselves. This can be something to take care of our mental, emotional, or physical health. Agnes Wanman once said, "Self-care is something that refuels us, rather than takes from us."

Does going to the bathroom alone refuel you? How about shopping alone for your family? How about going into your room to take a fifteen-minute power nap after being up all night with a colicky child?

The sad thing is many women might say yes. Those things do give you a boost. Yet the boost is more like a breather than restorative, long-lasting self-care.

What if we stopped calling activities self-care that don't bring joy or refuel?

In general, men are better at recognizing their own needs for self-care. My husband knows that mowing the yard alone isn't his self-care. Yes, maybe it feels a little nicer than being inside with three whiny kids, but it's still not self-care by his own definition.

Instead, he recognizes that his self-care is deliberately planning time for himself to do something physical like climbing mountains or going on a bike ride. It's intentional and planned out. It serves only him. And he's not multitasking in his mind twenty-three other things in the process. *I wish I could do that.*

What if we ask ourselves what we are actively doing to care for ourselves—something that has nothing to do with the rest of the people in our lives whom we serve at home or at work?

We should ask ourselves daily, *What am I doing that is intentional, planned out, and solely for me to refuel my mind, body, and soul?*

Then do what comes to mind. Make it happen. This is the type of care that supports your mental well-being and helps you to be a better mom, wife, friend, daughter, and overall human.

We need to take the time to sit with the reality that maybe we aren't caring for ourselves the way we really need it. If the fifteen-minute cup of coffee is what you love and feels restorative, then great!

But if you long for that girls' getaway and never take it because you feel too much guilt or don't have the means or support from your partner, try not to tell yourself that you only deserve that hot cup of joe and that's good enough.

If we pretend something is good enough but long for something more, it is damaging to our own mental and physical well-being. It's also sending the wrong message to those around us. Including our kids.

Your kids need to know what real self-care looks like.

If you ask your partner for a trip alone to the grocery store and you call it self-care, he's going to always think that's all you need to refuel and recharge and survive. But if you ask him to be in charge for a weekend and you truly come back recharged, then a higher standard is set. I am notorious for settling. The people pleaser in me doesn't want to inconvenience the entire world for a few days and nights alone.

Self-care is not going to fix all of life's problems. There may not be a fix to any of what you're going through, but giving yourself space is a way to allow yourself to breathe.

What Type of Self-Care Do You Need?

Consider these tips for helping you start to breathe again:

Make a self-care list.
The key here is to identify what will refuel you. Only you know that. When was the last time you asked yourself what you need, in order to take care of your mental, spiritual, and physical well-being? The thing that makes you feel like yourself, mind, body, and soul? Here is my list in no order.

- Broadway shows
- Girls' trips
- Writing
- Reality TV
- Keeping a running list of my strengths and my wins as a mom
- Therapy
- Getting back in bed occasionally when the kids are off to school
- Podcasts and books
- Exercise

- Time with my dog at the park
- Getting a babysitter for no reason at all
- Replacing every "I should" with "I can if I feel like it, but I don't have to"
- Locking myself in my room during the awful hour that is bedtime and letting my husband be in charge

Communicate with your support system.

It's much harder to get the kind of self-care you need without a support system. The amount of people with whom I must communicate to take a long weekend trip is kind of hysterical. Ok, here it goes.

First, I ask a neighbor to help with the dog and tell my carpool people. Second, I make sure our calendar is filled out correctly so that my husband can keep it all straight. I could go on and on.

Communicating with those in your circle who can help facilitate your self-care is important. If they don't know that you feel like a shell of a human being, how will they know to help?

Self-care is crucial to your survival as a mom. You've got this. Figure it out, and refuel the heck out of that soul of yours. Most importantly, give yourself grace.

CHAPTER 6

Loads of Grace

Giving ourselves grace can be hard when parts of motherhood are not fun or enjoyable. But giving ourselves grace can absolutely help lighten our mental load.

For example, like me, you probably underestimated the day-to-day annoying aspects of parenting. You know, things like walking into a room with an entire box of cereal spilled—or worse, cereal spilled *and* crushed—on the floor.

It's never really about the box of spilled cereal. It's more likely about the anxiety you're feeling because you're worried you aren't enough. Or about the shame you feel after an overreaction and your kids look at you with disappointment.

When you decide to have kids you don't think of all the daily stuff that quickly becomes overwhelming. Like the constant laundry and dishes and the kindergartener's calendar that would rival any CEO's. When did it become normal to keep an entire calendar dedicated to soccer matches, basketball games, ballet practice, and piano recitals . . . for a kindergartner? They can't even spell their last name, and they have more appointments on their calendars than the average adult!

You don't consider how draining it will be to walk around the house daily (most likely muttering something under your breath that begins with "Am I the only one who . . .") while putting away other people's stuff. Cleaning up messes. Trying to remember to switch the laundry and not forget that you're out of Ziploc gallon bags and your oldest has a book report due tomorrow.

I underestimated the repetitive nature of parenting. The repetition of my voice, reminders, tantrums, and arguments. Or how underwhelming it might feel to be the chauffeur for the big kids and try to keep everyone else busy, happy, and educated at the expense of myself.

I hadn't considered how something spilling on the floor at the end of the day (that's really *so easy* to clean up) might push me over the edge.

I never considered all the noise and how cranky I would be.

In all seriousness, everyday annoyances can feel suffocating. That's what the mental load is like for me. It's the annoyances in between the joyful moments that drag me down.

It's the adulting and being responsible for all the things.

Parenting can be boring and annoying and lame and overwhelming and miserable. There, I said it. Sometimes, being a mom can be miserable.

Wait a minute. Hear me out.

I write a lot of mom jokes online about the struggles of motherhood. I share the hard stuff so I will laugh and not cry. A woman left a response to a funny tongue-in-cheek meme I wrote as I vented about the struggles of parenting. She simply said, "I never want to be a mom because it sounds miserable."

It *does* sound miserable sometimes. That's because it absolutely can be.

- There are hard things we don't know how to deal with.
- Some kids suffer because of bullying, friendship problems, and heartbreak.
- Husbands and kids can be unappreciative on days when you've put your heart and soul into mothering.
- Kids can talk back and say they hate you.
- Stomach bugs can hit the whole house at the worst possible time.
- Kids remember book reports at the last minute, and you stay up until midnight when you just want to sleep, and babies become crazy sleepless monsters just when they started sleeping five hours straight.

Beyond that there are harder things, like when your son struggles with debilitating school anxiety and you know he gets that from you. We went through a rough patch where my son was refusing to go to school and I had no clue how to help him. I knew it was a manifestation of his anxiety, but I felt helpless.

Some Days You Won't Know What You're Doing

There are times when you feel like you don't know what you're doing—because you don't.

There are times when you feel like you're failing everything and everyone.

I'll never forget the year when my middle child was in preschool. I was so proud of another one of my kiddos finally being out in the world; I also had one in kindergarten doing so well and a newborn baby. But this middle child would *not* be the forgotten one. Middle children in my house will never be forgotten. I was up to my eyeballs trying to do all the things. I was a mom learning how to navigate being in the PTA and how the public school system worked. I was working from home with my budding writing career and nursing a colicky newborn.

No worries. I am woman, hear me roar! Right? I would do it all. I would never drop the ball. My middle child would never be forgotten.

Until he was.

It was a rare bright and balmy morning when I seemingly had all my crap together. I swear to you I was convinced I was nailing this motherhood gig. The baby was fed and had a clean diaper, and the oldest was off to school. Only a few minutes left until I got my full two and a half glorious hours of time when my middle was also out of the house and it was just me and the baby running a lot of errands.

I was standing in the kitchen totally nailing mother-hood and being a badass, and I heard a tiny voice behind me say something about dress-up day at school.

It was as if a record scratched.

"Dress-up day? What are you talking about?"

"We're supposed to dress up as what we want to be when we 'gwow' up. For 'caweer' day." *What the heck?* I thought to myself looking nervously at the clock. Career day.

Did I see a note about this? Did he tell me and I forgot? We have approximately 5.8 minutes until we need to be driving in the car to get to preschool for my well-deserved two and a half hours of one-kid-only shopping time, and dammit I need this to work out. Think, *Meredith!*

I smiled cheerfully to the big baby blue eyes looking up at me. "I want to be Batman."

"Batman isn't a career!" *Think, Meredith. What costumes do we have that can be a career?*

"How about a doctor?" I tried to act enthusiastic even though I could see the joy draining from my little boy's face right in front of me.

"But I don't want to be a doctor." He started pouting.

I ignored the sweet cherub (that I promised never to ignore because of middle child syndrome), and I grabbed a white button-down shirt from my husband's closet because it looked like a lab coat. Then I grabbed his stetho-scope and old magnetic name tag from PA school. Voila! We had a doctor.

I threw the preschooler and the baby in the car, and we were on our way. *I'm a rockstar*, I thought to myself. Can you believe what I just pulled off? I pulled together a career day costume in 4.7 seconds, and he's still going to be on time. I proudly drove all the way to preschool thinking I was superhuman.

I pulled up to his preschool, and when my son got out we saw another kid dressed as—you guessed it—Batman. Then it hit me. I had screwed up. Why did I care if he was Batman for career day? Batman was badass. He saved people, and he would win in a battle against Spiderman, and I'm pretty sure he has a giant mansion in Gotham City, so it's got to be a career or something.

My son was none the wiser and enjoyed his career day, but I felt like a total and complete failure. It was miserable.

So yes, motherhood can feel terrible some days. We're going to screw up and make mistakes and disappoint our kids. It's inevitable.

Motherhood Can Also Be Miserable in the Best Possible Way

With all the misery we sometimes feel while mothering, there are big rewards that make it so worth it.

- You wonder why you did this to yourself but are reminded when you get an unsolicited thank you from your hormonal teenager.
- You wonder if you are cut out for any of it, but then you realize you are—when your first grader does

something kinder than you would have done in the same situation.

- You get snuggles and hugs and a fierce unconditional love that lasts forever.
- You get laughs and inside jokes with little people who really are your best friends.
- You get companionship for life and the satisfaction of watching another human discover things in the world.
- You see yourself in them—both the good and the bad—and you are proud that they are yours.

The mental load of motherhood is the kind of misery that fosters growth, patience, love, and grace—all things that make up a good human being.

I never considered the joy I could feel watching another human discover and experience life. That's why it's so hard to explain parenting to someone who hasn't lived it. You underestimate so much. The good, the bad, the terrible. The feelings and emotions and the mundane. It's all a big fat beautiful mess that we love and hate all in the same day but wouldn't trade for anything. The love is too big.

What you get in return can't be summed up in words—as much as the writer in me hates that fact. It's the kind of misery that brings inexplicable joy with it and unexpected gifts you didn't know you needed.

Despite this constant back-and-forth between misery and joy, on some days it just feels like you can't do it.

Give Yourself Grace on the Days When It Feels Impossible

How do you give yourself grace when you forget to see joy in day-to-day life? How do you give yourself grace when that mental load takes over and you can't get out of bed?

I had a depressive episode for about a year, and I had a hard time getting out of bed most days.

There were so many times when the urge to lie in bed was so strong, I didn't think I could keep going. I would force myself to get up for my kids in the morning. Some days, I believe that it was solely because of them that I survived. Difficult to admit, but true.

It was hard to be there for them, but it was also good for me to have something to do. Some sort of responsibility to get me out of bed in the mornings. Did I dread the morning routines of getting them off to school? Yes. Did I occasionally go right back to bed after they left? Also yes.

Although the anxiety of raising kids is an obstacle to overcome, I find that it allows me time to grow in a way I didn't expect. The constant screw-ups that I make as a mother are frequently difficult to accept. I get angry. I yell. I feel like my kids deserve so much more. I have to fight those feelings daily while in the trenches of mundane chores that make up running a household. I have to give myself grace in the little and the big things. Still, I have some days that I call my "I can't" days.

"I Can't" Days

Some days just seem impossible to get through. From the moment I open my eyes, I'm dreaming about one thing only: closing them again in the evening.

The last time I had an "I can't" day, I stared into space and attempted a nap that didn't really pan out.

I went on a walk in the morning—my usual routine—and I was S-L-O-W. It was a stroll, y'all. My legs felt like tree trunks, and I swear my dog dragged me up the hill near my house. A grandma with a walker could have passed me, and I wouldn't have noticed.

It wasn't much in the way of vigorous exercise, but hey, at least I got out.

Those days are hard. And when I have them, I just keep hearing the words in my head: "I can't."

It's not a cop-out, although it can certainly feel like it. On "I can't" days, I physically do not have the energy. And I usually don't have the emotional energy either.

I will feel like I'm slipping into depression again. It's a scary feeling because you can almost see it coming. You can see the storm rolling in from the distance.

What's weird is that "I can't" days can also come out of the blue. They are typically followed by days when my brain is in overdrive and I need more hours in the day to accomplish all the ideas that are coming into my head. Then it will feel like my soul is sucked out of me. And it's not even my kids doing it this time.

When I become an "I can't" person, it feels so frustrating.

Some people don't like the negative connotation of words like "I can't," but when you suffer from depression or anxiety, those words just feel true. Even if they're not.

I also have days when I can. I will have tons of energy. I will be happy. I am optimistic on the "I can" days. I make the phone calls I've been putting off and check off the to-do list with enthusiasm. Sometimes I even text my husband and list everything I've done because I'm so proud of my productivity. The days when I'm in over-drive accomplishing everything, feel euphoric. I wish I had those days every day. But, the "I can't" days still come back, unfortunately.

I had a fifth-grade teacher who was super diligent about directing us away from saying "can" or "can't" when we asked for something. "Ms. Jensen?" I would raise my hand. "Can I go to the bathroom?"

She would smile with a twinkle in her eye and say, "I don't know—*can* you?" I think of her when I say, "I can't." I can almost hear her asking, "Is that true, Meredith? Or can you?"

When you struggle with mental illness or the mother load or anxiety, your mental limitations make the "I can't" so much stronger.

Sometimes your brain just can't in those moments. Or that's what your brain is telling you.

It keeps you from feeling like you can put one foot in front of the other.

It keeps you from feeling like you can have a clear thought, or you feel confused.

It keeps you from feeling like there's a point to yard work and laundry, or cooking a healthy meal.

Technically, you're still doing it.

I used to feel bad about my "I can't" days.

Now I give myself grace in those moments and accept the "I can't" days. On those days, I recognize that I did a lot of things.

True, it probably took me longer.

I was slower.

I was foggier.

I wasn't exactly cheerful or happy.

I didn't enjoy it.

I maybe even resented it.

I may have even spent time sitting and doing nothing.

But I still did a lot of things.

The point in giving ourselves grace when we're having a day like this is not to count all our accomplishments. The point is that if we can give ourselves grace on the "I can't" days, then technically we still can.

It's OK if we aren't on overdrive. It's OK if we stare into space or wear sweats to the store and walk around like a zombie. We're still at the store, mama! We're doing it.

We are accomplishing and still functional—not as quickly and as beautifully as we accomplish things on the other days, perhaps, but that's not the point. The point is, we are fighting the part of us that tells us we can't—and—giving ourselves grace at the same time.

Let's be honest. There are days when not doing anything is all you can do. So if you have "I can't" days too, you're still good, worthy, important, and valuable. It was just a day. You got through it.

That means you *can* do something. And you did.

Mothering in day-to-day life looks like a lot of hard work. It looks like making choices that seem simple to others all while we are fighting our brain's negative feelings about ourselves all day long. Give yourself all the grace. Let your kids know you're having an off day. They will give grace to you too. They will also learn it's important to give grace to themselves as well.

Allow yourself grace to move through the world at a different pace.

And you'll see, by giving yourself grace in those challenges that are little (and big), that the next day and its grueling to-do lists will seem more manageable.

Before you know it, you'll have done it for a solid eighteen years and realize it was worth it . . . every miserable, breathtaking, heart-warming, life-changing moment.

SECTION TWO

Society's Little Lies

Mothers have martyred themselves in their children's names since the beginning of time. We have lived as if she who disappears the most, loves the most. We have been conditioned to prove our love by slowly ceasing to exist. **—Glennon Doyle, *Untamed***

CHAPTER 7

Everything Is Awesome!

When my oldest came along I had high hopes. I was not going to yell. I was not going to lose my patience. I certainly wasn't going to have negative thoughts. Nope. Not me. No way. *Shudder*.

Motherhood was going to be all rainbows and story time, giggles, hugs, cuddles, I love you's, patience, and matching Christmas pajamas.

When my first child was born, my husband was in graduate school and started his surgery rotation the next day. He left me in the hospital as a brand-new mom with this squirmy little creature, and he took our only car and drove an hour away to meet with the doctor he would be working under for the next six weeks.

Thankfully, the doctor sent him home that day after realizing we had just had our first child the night before. But in the days that followed, I was left at home in our tiny two-bedroom apartment in Philadelphia with no car, no family close by, and really no friends. This was before Facebook and smartphones were a thing and you could interact with people all day online. Instead, I was bleeding and crying into the milk gushing from my watermelon-sized breasts.

My only outlet was scrapbooking, and I would work for hours between feedings to carefully control the papers and ribbons so they created elaborate pages of color documenting every little coo and sweet smile that happened with my new baby. We went on walks to the park, but I didn't live in an area with a lot of young mothers. I lived in an area with a lot of concrete and urban apartments where people worked during the day. I felt isolated and alone. I cried every single day. For months.

The worst part of those first few months wasn't necessarily the leaky boobs or the isolation; it was the fear. The absolute fear I wasn't doing any of it right because it didn't feel like I had imagined. Where were the good parts of all of this? Motherhood was not what I had expected. What had I done to myself? Why did I decide to become a mother? Was I already screwing it up?

There was certainly no one to vent to, minus my sister, who always understood. She was my lifeline, and I am convinced that every mother needs a friend or a support system during their motherhood journey. Because, in my mind, new motherhood was something you treasured and enjoyed and basked in, and I needed her to reassure me on those hard days.

You certainly weren't supposed to cry every day of motherhood. I knew that much.

I was determined I had to get it right and if I didn't, I would ruin my baby, myself, or my relationship with my husband. At least that's what I had convinced myself with my pre-kid expectations of motherhood.

I would wake up constantly those first few months to check on her. She slept right next to me, and I didn't sleep a wink.

I was obsessed with watching her little chest move up and down at night to make sure she didn't die. I just knew it might happen on my watch, and I was determined not to screw up. I would do it absolutely flawlessly. The sleep, the feedings, the mothering. Everything.

It was all-consuming in a way that suffocated me, and I didn't even realize what was happening because I had this beautiful creature in front of me smiling and making cute faces. I was in *love*.

But I felt like I wasn't getting it right. It certainly didn't feel wonderful.

I tried to sleep when the baby slept, but obsessive thoughts filled my mind:

Is she sleeping too long?

It's too quiet.

What was that noise?

Did she get enough at her last feeding?

What if she cries and I don't hear her?

Is she eating and growing enough?

If she moved a little in her sleep, maybe it was SIDS. If she didn't move in her sleep, maybe it was SIDS.

I did not nap those first few months unless she was in my arms, and even then, I was terrified of dropping her or rolling over her.

My anxiety enabled me to imagine terrifying scenarios such as tripping when I was holding her or forgetting to check on her. I became hypervigilant. I had a hard time letting my husband do anything because I was so worried something bad would happen.

I couldn't let her out of my sight without panicking, and I was terrified to leave the house *with* her.

In fact, my first postpartum trip to the store alone, she hated her car seat and cried—no, screamed—the entire fifteen-minute drive. I tried to remain calm, but I knew I was committing an egregious act against this small child by daring to go to Target to pick up a few things and feel somewhat normal. I turned the car around minutes before arriving at Target and went home. At this point, we were both crying.

I didn't tell anyone about all these intrusive thoughts I was having, imagining every worst-case scenario. Because they were ugly. And dark. And scary.

What kind of mother imagines the worst thing happening to her baby all the time?

After four months of anguished crying every day, I remember vividly the day a light broke through the clouds. My daughter found her thumb and started sleeping long stretches at night, and for the first day since giving birth, I didn't cry. It was eye-opening. I realized for the first time that I was suffering from postpartum depression and anxiety. And it was finally lifting.

I became happier and a little more confident in my abilities. I was finally able to get some sleep, which I'm sure directly correlated to my ability to be happy and confident.

Yet the nagging thought in my mind that I wasn't doing it right never completely left me. Society told me motherhood is so wonderful. But it certainly didn't feel that way when I was depressed.

It's a lie my mind continues to tell me even now due to the conditioning I've received, the impossible societal standards, and the constant in-your-face Instagram moms:

I will never get it right.
I'm not a good mom.
This doesn't feel wonderful.
Everything is not awesome.

I realized society has it all wrong. Motherhood isn't always so wonderful.

It certainly isn't awesome all the time.

I'd love to be the guy from the Lego movie walking around singing, "Everything is awesome!" at the top of my lungs, but the truth is, motherhood can have days where nothing is awesome.

> **Motherhood isn't always so wonderful.**

That's a lie society tells us. Motherhood can suck. Sometimes we're depressed. And there are times we don't feel like a good mom.

It's Normal to Feel Like You're Not a Good Mom

The tireless task of mothering and the impossible task of feeling like you need to always get it right creates a mental mess where you feel like a failure every day. A mother constantly fights against the toxic thoughts that she should be doing it better, different, or more gracefully.

Let me give you an example.

A couple of years ago, I reached the point where all three of my kids were in school all day long, but all I felt was pain and regret. I had been looking forward to having the house to myself for years. Literally. I'm pretty sure it was something I would daydream about during midnight feedings and temper tantrums.

It felt impossibly far away when I was in the trenches.

Instead of celebrating my newfound kid-free hours of freedom, I sat around worrying I had missed the best parts of their little kid years. My kids were no longer babies, and what if I hadn't enjoyed it enough? What if I'd wasted it away working, or staring at my phone, or doing laundry, or just saying no instead of giving my kids yes days?

I suddenly had hours of alone time, and I was completely and utterly lost for a few weeks. I would dare say I was even depressed. Why was I like this? Why couldn't I just be proud that we had moved on to the next stage of life devoid of diapers and preschoolers?

But eventually those feelings passed, and I was busier than ever. I found my way back to the business of taking care of my work, a home, and the entire family.

Moving into a new stage of parenting can sometimes hurt if we don't recognize that we're doing the best we can in each moment.

There was one night during the elementary years when

my daughter wanted to play a game as a family. Sounds like good family fun, right?

Well, my children turned into wild monkey-like versions of themselves after consuming a few calories, and they started acting feral.

Instead of sitting down to play the game, I sent them outside where they could run and scream. I was hoping they would expend the pent-up energy. One could argue that I was a good mom for seeing they needed exercise.

Yet my flawed mom brain still argued I wasn't a good mom during this stage either because I didn't have the patience to calm them down enough to play Uno. They just come home from school, so why was I already annoyed with them?

No matter what my circumstances were, I never felt like I was measuring up. If they were home with me as toddlers, I was failing. If they were gone to school all day and then I sent them outside to play, I was failing.

Feeling like you're constantly in fail mode is painful. It's normal to feel like you're not a good mom, but it's not good for you. Constantly feeling stuck in fail mode will make you look back on your parenting with regrets instead of realizing you enjoyed so much of the journey.

What If We Could Love the Mothers We Actually Are?

I have loved my kids with a vengeance since the moment I laid eyes on them. The hardest part for me is learning to love myself.

Like many moms, I fall into the trap of believing that if it doesn't feel awesome all the time, the motherhood experience isn't wonderful and—worse—I'm not a good mom.

I love this quote from one of my favorite podcasts[5]—which I think about often in the context of mothering: "What screws us up most in life is the picture in our head of how it's supposed to be." We should never judge our parenting based on our pre-kid expectations of ourselves. Instead, we need to love the parents we are. Our kids certainly do. So why shouldn't we?

We feel like our kids deserve someone better.

What if we decided though to love ourselves radically as imperfect moms? What if we looked in the mirror and, instead of being disappointed, said out loud, "I'm a good mom most of the time. And that's perfectly OK."

What if instead of singing, "Everything is awesome!" we sang something more realistic, such as, "Everything's not awesome. But I'll make it through today anyway. Everything's not awesoooome!"

Who defines what a perfect mom looks like anyway? Is it a mom who never yells? Or a mom who only uses cloth diapers? Is it the mom who never takes a break?

If you stop to break down what the "perfect" mom looks like, you'll realize she was never meant to exist.

Our definition of a good mom needs to morph into something a tad more realistic. It needs to include the messy parts of human nature like occasional anger and frustration along with the beautiful parts like love and forgiveness.

Our children only need us to show up in our own

humanity to be perfect for them. That's how they learn it's safe to show up in their own humanity and imperfectness.

They need connection, safety, and love. That's it.

Providing those basic needs to our kids will allow them space to show up messy as well and build healthy connections as they grow that are flawed, but beautiful.

So how do we start to learn to love ourselves?

Look out for yourself.

This goes back to taking care of yourself. Practicing the self-care that really rejuvenates you and makes you feel good.

Look at yourself the way you'd look at a mama friend.

You're not criticizing her every decision, so why are you doing this to yourself? Try accepting your flaws the way you'd accept a friend's flaws. Offer encouraging words to yourself like you'd offer your bestie.

A friend of mine once told me that her daughter picked up on her negative self-thoughts and said, "Mom, I wish you could see yourself the way I see you. I wish you could borrow my eyes to see what I see." It was simple yet profound. It was a turning point for her to change the way she thought of herself and begin to practice self-love in front of her daughter, because she wants that for her daughter.

Love yourself the way you want your kids to love themselves.

We are our own worst critics. That's universal. We don't want to pass along this idea to our kids—that they're never good enough—by constantly tearing ourselves down.

Whether our kids notice us doing this overtly or it's solely an internal struggle that brings you down, loving and accepting your own imperfect mothering every single day is modeling true self-love to your kids. They need to love themselves with a vengeance, and so do you.

Radically loving the mom you already are, so you can pour that love, safety, and connection into your kids is the key to finding peace in the journey and noticing what really makes motherhood awesome.

CHAPTER 8

Just Wash Your Face, and It Will Be OK

Not too long ago, a book came out that was *flying* off the shelves.

Everyone was talking about it. I felt icky inside whenever I thought about the title. The whole premise of the book just felt off to me.

Solve your problems by washing your face? Ummmm . . . excuse me?

Now, don't get me wrong. It was a bestseller, and people ate it up. The message obviously worked for some people. But I knew as soon as I heard the title that the message was not going to be for me.

I decided right then I was going to write a book called *Girl, Don't Shower for Days.* I'll admit the title didn't really work. There was a chance I could have gotten sued. It bothered me that some women who desperately needed a message of solidarity and empathy in their dark times were instead getting a message that they were in control of their own destiny and if they would just try harder, it would all be OK. Everything in my soul rebelled at the thought.

You can only fix what you can control, and life is full of stuff you cannot control, fix, or predict. Things just happen to us that no amount of face washing is going to fix. And honestly? There are times when you just need to let your face stay dirty.

One day happened when I was a young mom to two kids. I had gone on an outing with my mom, my three-year-old, and the baby, who was probably about five months at the time. I have no idea where we went or what we were doing, but I remember that as I was rounding the corner to my street, I was daydreaming about putting kids down for naps and having a minute to myself.

I swear, if there were a Mom Fairy who flew around granting wishes, her main job would be waving her wand to put all our kids down for a nap at the same time. The gift of being able to rest my eyes for a minute and hearing my own thought without Elmo singing in the background would be better than a dollar bill under my pillow, any day.

On the drive home, it started to rain. Like, a large, Georgia-style rainstorm. Even if you try to make a dash from your driveway to the front door, you still end up looking like the girl climbing out of a well from *The Ring*.

As I drove, I heard and smelled something from the backseat. My nostrils stung. The baby. He was grunting and squirming, and a big shart erupted throughout the car.

He had one of those poops. A watery, breastfeeding poop. Not only could I smell the familiar smell of yellow poo, but I could feel in my bones that it was bad. Call it mother's intuition; I just knew it was the kind that all moms dread.

You know, the kind that shoots up their back like Old Faithful and squirts out every opening in their clothing. Yep, it was exactly that kind. A bath was needed ASAP. I needed to take the whole car seat with me, because you know it was covered.

I started calculating how we were going to make this work. Mom and I had to get a preschooler down for a nap and a baby inside quickly while navigating the pouring rain and poopmageddon in the backseat.

I pulled into our long driveway and hit the garage door button. Something darted out.

Meeeeoooooow! But it sounded more like a horrifying woodland creature from an M. Night Shyamalan movie.

OMG. The cat. I just ran over the cat.

Wait. Did I say that out loud?

"Mommy? Is kitty OK?" I heard from my three-year-old in the backseat.

Ohhh no. I did say it out loud. I reassured her that kitty was fine, wondering how much a lie like that would cost later in therapy dollars.

What do I do? Do I pull forward? Do I back up? Is the cat mangled under the tire? I didn't see her run off anywhere after she screeched.

After running through every possible scenario in my mind in a matter of 2.3 seconds, I decided the best decision was to back up in case she was stuck under the tire.

I put the car in reverse, and the worst thing happened. I heard the noise again.

Meeeeooooow!

I burst into tears. I'm sure my mom was trying to console me through all of this, but I have no recollection of her saying anything back to me as I shouted, "Oh my gosh! I just killed the cat!"

My oldest started to cry in the backseat. The baby started crying too. I didn't dare move the car again because the cat was for sure dead. I heard my mom say, "Why don't you just take the kids inside? I'll find the cat."

When I got out of the car, the cat was thankfully not a pancake on my driveway. She was gone. Whether this was a blessing or a curse, I did not know.

I took the kids inside in a mad, wet dash, and I called my husband at work, hysterical.

"I ran over the cat. And now she's in the woods somewhere dying." My daughter was looking at me with wide saucer eyes.

My husband, bless his heart, came home and spent thirty minutes stomping through the muddy woods, searching for the remains of our family pet in a torrential downpour. He came back empty-handed, and whatever hope I had left drained out of me.

That was it. I had killed the cat.

My child's first pet got run over by her mother.

Talk about feeling low. It was the lowest.

After all children were settled and bathed, my husband returned to work, and I was finally able to calm down, I heard something at the back door.

It was a little tiny scratch.

The cat was back.

And she was totally freaking fine.

Not a scratch or a limp.

After all that, I was honestly a little pissed she was alive.

Maybe the whole nine lives business is real and our cat hadn't been playing fast and loose with her other lives. Maybe I ran over someone else's cat.

Things Just Happen to Us

We are never able to control it all, and as a result, we can't always just have a better attitude and pick ourselves up by the bootstraps to fix things.

For example, maybe your kid threw up all night, or you just lost your job.

Perhaps you're getting a divorce, after investing in a fifteen-year relationship. Or you don't know how you're going to pay your bills this week.

Maybe the toddler is in the terrible twos and making life hell, or maybe you're estranged from your family and you don't know how to fix it, or you just got out of an abusive relationship.

It could be you recently lost a child, a best friend, or a spouse. *Nothing* can fix that. Nothing.

The problem with the whole washing-your-face platitude or picking-yourself-up-by-the-bootstraps mentality is that both create this idea that any failure you have is your personal responsibility.

Hard things just happen to us. A lot of the chaos that ensued from the cat incident just happened. The rainstorm. The cat darting underneath the car. That unbelievable baby bowel explosion.

None of those things were because of my personal failure. It was just a really bad day. Yet I felt responsible in some way for all of it.

If your best friend described that day to you and she felt like a failure for any of it, you would reassure her that you love her and it is not her fault. We have an easier time giving grace to others.

> **We have an easier time giving grace to others.**

If you buy into the idea that your ability to be a good mom is based on how smoothly your day goes, I have news for you: the cat may dart under the car when you least expect it.

You can't feel like a bad mom because things aren't working out the way you planned.

Not Only Do Things Happen to Us, But They Often Aren't Fixable

You can't unpancake the cat in the driveway or unpoop the diaper blowout that ruins your favorite sweater. I was just pulling into my driveway, dreaming of naptime, minding my own business, when all hell broke loose.

Thankfully, the cat was fine, and she's now fourteen years old and as crabby and psycho as ever. But if she had died, would I have been able to fix it for my child?

Would telling her to quickly wash her face or pull herself together have erased her pain of losing her first pet?

Washing your face doesn't allow you the chance to sit in grief and pain.

It doesn't allow for personal growth.

Can we normalize *not* picking ourselves up right away to cope with the cat we just ran over accidentally? Can we normalize letting ourselves sit in pain and grief and trauma sometimes? Can we normalize that life is full of struggles (and so is parenting)?

If you're struggling right now and not feeling super positive about things, it's OK.

There is still hope. Life, motherhood, and the daily grind is not as easy as washing your face and bucking up. I wish it were.

It's about relying on a friend to carry you.

It's about allowing yourself to feel all the hard stuff so that when it's over, the joy will be that much sweeter.

It's about finding your people—even when a simple smile from a stranger in the grocery store is what helps you put one foot in front of the other.

It's about being part of humanity; we are meant to lift each other up, not just do it all alone.

Yes, you've got this.

You've got this because people everywhere are willing to help you push through the hard stuff.

Don't feel like showering for days? We won't judge you, because that's life. There are days when you just can't wash your face, and that's OK.

CHAPTER 9

You Can Have It All.
#BossBabe

My definition of having it all has changed multiple times throughout my evolution as a mother. When I first heard the phrase, "You can have it all," I thought it meant you were supposed to have a career, raise perfect kids, keep a clean house, have nonstop sex with your husband, stay skinny, and volunteer as PTA president too.

It only took having one kid for me to realize no one is a superhuman, and having it all sounded downright exhausting to be a boss babe. So I decided having it all must really mean we had to bask in motherhood and find joy in whatever our circumstances were.

Maybe we'd count our blessings, and then we would *feel* like we had it all.

I tricked myself into believing I shouldn't want more than what I already had. I had a good husband, a modest and comfortable home, three kids, and the ability to stay home with them.

I even wrote a blog post about five or six years ago about how having it all was possible if we could adjust the lens we see through.

My takeaway of that blog post was that you simply have to find the joy. That's it. That's the whole key to having it all. Sounds easy enough, right?

I look back at "my life was meant to be joy-full" mindset from that blog post, and I see the struggle I was wrestling with. I was trying to tell myself to be grateful and not want anything at all.

Yikes.

I'm still a big believer of gratitude, but I don't think having it all is as simple as adopting a Pollyanna attitude.

I Don't Know If It's Possible to Have It All

Years ago, I was walking the aisles of World Market for no reason and saw a sign that caught my eye. It was black and white and metal and went with my aesthetic—black and white—and I knew I had to have it.

The sign simply said,

Every Cloud Has a Silver Lining

I was sold. I knew this was going to be my new mantra. I looked at that sign and thought, *This is a good message.* This is something I need hanging in my home to remind me to look for the good in every situation. This will help me "find the joy."

Looking for the good in every situation was mostly out of character for me, but I must have been feeling particularly optimistic that day. I'm a glass-half-empty kind of girl. Raised by an eternal pessimist I learned to look for the opposite of the silver lining in every situation.

So clearly, this sign was absolutely what I needed hanging in my home. Plus, like everything in World Market, it was cute.

My husband must have thought I lost my marbles when I proudly hung that sign in our dining room because, well, he knew me. He knew I was a glass-half-empty kind of girl, definitely not an "Every cloud has a silver lining" kind of girl.

That sign has faded into the background of my home décor. I hardly notice it anymore. I looked at it recently and realized the saying was not helping anyone.

I'm not sure it ever helped at all, really. Keep that in mind when you see those cute Rae Dunn signs at Home Goods. I promise, you don't need another inspirational sign, my friends.

It's whimsical and idealistic, sure. But is it making me see the silver lining in my everyday life? Am I finding the joy in all the moments? Do I have it all?

Nah.

The Times When Gratitude and Silver Linings Aren't Enough

I realized about a year ago that by searching for a silver lining in everything, I was invalidating my feelings and the feelings of those around me.

And that didn't sit well with me.

When we try to pull out a silver lining moment amid something like a pandemic, it falls flat. Our intention is usually good but misguided.

At the beginning of the pandemic, I remember people trying to put a silver lining around what was happening. Meanwhile people were dying by the thousands.

I, like so many others, was asking myself terrifying questions like, *Do I need to wipe down my groceries with Clorox wipes and wait to put them away until the germs are gone?* It was scary.

The last thing I wanted to hear was something like, "At least we're not spending money eating out so much!"

Yet I heard so many things like that. It was its own type of virus spreading across social media.

When high-school seniors couldn't graduate in person, people would say, "At least you can do a Zoom graduation!"

Mothers everywhere were thrust into homeschooling. I would see experienced homeschooling moms diminish others' struggles by saying, "It's not like it's hard! We've been doing it for years!"

You didn't dare lament anything, because you would immediately be told to be grateful you weren't dying.

I'm glad in some ways we came together in our collective suffering for a little while, though it seemed there was more vitriol than compassion in the comments section.

I *do* think gratitude can help us shift our perspective and appreciate what we have. And looking for silver linings can be a positive thing, unless it is used as weapon, in which case it can make others feel incredibly alone. Some may not even realize they are dismissing others' pain by introducing alternative ways of thinking. Sometimes it is best to allow the person to be in the moment, just listen, and be there for her.

"Having it all" doesn't mean that we just sugar coat the hard parts, feel gratitude, and look for the positive. For me, having it all means that we accept it ALL—the ugly parts of life and the pretty ones. It's going through our mothering

> I *do* think gratitude can help us shift our perspective and appreciate what we have.

journey realizing that sometimes we screw up, sometimes we succeed, and we're all living life messy, and that's OK.

Having It All Means Something Different to Everyone

I've finally landed on the idea that having it all means I'm living an authentic life and accepting all that entails.

It means stepping into my own, listening to myself, and doing what works best for me and my family. Having it all should not come from a checklist that society has told us makes us successful. It's a state of mind. Are we living life to the fullest with our own unique skills and talents? Are we listening to the needs of our children or watching what other moms are doing on social media? Are we closing the books about parenting and trusting our gut? Are we embracing what makes us unique and living our life in a way that is meaningful and supports that uniqueness? Doing what works best for you and your family is key to having it all.

Society lies to us that having it all means we must get things just right as a mom to be good at it. We must have a career and raise amazing kids and do all the other stuff that makes up the life of being an adult to have it all.

For me, having it all means knowing yourself. Loving her. And letting her lead the way.

How Can You Find Out What Having It All Looks Like to You?

We have to step into ourselves.

Live an authentic life
that is unique to you. Don't be afraid to be yourself, even if it goes against everything you thought you knew about yourself. Embrace the changes that come naturally to you as you age. Remind yourself what makes you tick outside of motherhood.

Create your own checklist.
Don't worry about someone else's checklist or try to replicate someone else's life. We have no idea what that mom deals with behind the picture-perfect scenes. To another mom, having it all might mean a career, two kids, and volunteering at the PTA. Some women can do that. But are you focusing on your checklist or on the list of someone whom you perceive is put together more perfectly than you?

Get comfortable with what works for you and your family. Even if it looks different from everyone else. Remember that you can create what having it all means to you and then be OK if it doesn't always work out the way you planned. Accept that what works for you and your family might look messy to an outsider.

Maybe not having it all, as society defines it, is a gift. Because that's when we can slow down and say—*this is what it looks like to ME to have it all.*

CHAPTER 10

You Were Made for This

How many times have you heard the trope that motherhood will come naturally to you? I have heard it a million times, yet I felt like I was failing at motherhood before I even began. Yes, I loved my daughter as soon as she was put in my arms, but I also felt like motherhood was a little foreign to me. There was nothing "natural" about it.

And, no, I didn't feel made for this.

Some things I instinctively knew how to do, like feed my babies, change their diapers, and make sure they were soothed when crying. I figured out how to breastfeed fairly easily, and I knew how to hold my babies to make them feel comfortable.

Most mothers can do those things. So sure, in that sense motherhood comes naturally to all of us. We quickly understand a cry means x, y, or z, and you don't put a baby on the couch unsupervised if she can roll over on her own.

But being thrust into becoming a mother the instant you push a baby out of the aching, swollen, foreign-feeling body you've been waddling around in for nine months feels anything but natural. Sure, we got the baby here, that part our bodies knew how to do, but how does becoming a mother overnight shift instantly in our psyches?

Newsflash, it doesn't.

Becoming a Mother Overnight Is a Lot

Suddenly, your entire universe shifts when that baby comes. Your sleep schedule is garbage, your meal schedule involves small bites you can grab in between feeding your infant, and your whole world revolves around this tiny human who doesn't really give you much feedback on how you're doing.

It can feel suffocating to be a new mother.

I felt suffocated by the responsibility in my new role. Being a mom did not feel natural at all. How was it that I was now responsible for another human who needed so much? And before you think I was a young mom, I was twenty-nine years old! Part of me still didn't feel like an adult, much less an adult who was responsible for keeping another human alive and teaching that human literally everything. It was overwhelming.

Accepting my role as a mother took years.

Sixteen years in, I am surprised by the responsibility of it all. I'm even annoyed by it some days. (It's *natural* to feel *that* way.) We are human, and while we love our babies intensely, we also love ourselves. Human nature is inherently selfish. It takes years and years of practice to be good at sacrificing our own needs and desires for those of other people.

When you grow up in a family, you have to bend to the wants and desires of siblings or other family members. You learn as a toddler to do what your parents say instead of what you want.

Then you have to make adjustments in preschool, elementary, and high school that help you learn to compromise and work with others. And that continues when you're in college; you adjust to living with roommates and doing what they want and need to coexist.

In the workplace, you adjust to rules, schedules, and a boss's demands. Most jobs won't allow you to take a nap whenever you want.

When you get married, you compromise constantly about things like how to load the dishwasher, budget money, and so on. If you were alone, you'd probably do it how *you* like it, but when you're living with another person, you sacrifice what you want all the time. My husband and I have been joyfully married twenty years, and we still compromise daily.

Letting go of your own desires for the wants and needs of someone else is not a new concept. It is part of the human experience in every way.

Yet when women become mothers, suddenly they are expected to be naturally and immediately good at it.

We should be totally OK with shifting our entire world to this other human being because it's natural, right? You're supposed to love it. Society tells us we were made to birth babies and that's our purpose. But making that shift does not mean we're going to jump in and love it right away.

Good News: It's Not Always Natural

I'm here to tell you that it's ridiculous to think it's all going to be "natural" to give up sleep, adjust standards of living, wear clean clothes that don't smell of sour milk, and change our eating habits.

Oh, and it's fine that suddenly our partner is the last of our concerns because we have this new person in our life who is helpless. How is it supposed to feel natural to shift our focus to someone new whom we don't know yet? Not to mention that little person is a helpless, squishy, poop machine who can't even smile yet.

So why aren't we happy?

We haven't even touched on the fact many of us came from neglectful, abusive, or unstable homes. Some of us have detached mothers or absent fathers. It's highly possible we never experienced "natural motherhood"; we don't even know what natural motherhood looks like because the version we saw was not great.

It's OK to Admit It Does Not Come Naturally

I loved the newborn stage with my kids because the expectations were clear. Feed them, burp them, change them, and try your best to get them to sleep. It's when they became more independent, I started to realize I had no idea if I was doing any of it right.

I started to ask myself questions like, *What is the "right" choice that will do the least amount of damage to my kids? What do I do the first time they lie? How about when they say, "I hate you"? What if I lose my patience and yell? Are they damaged forever?*

With a three-month-old, I totally could limp along and figure it out; with a strong-willed four-year-old, I wasn't sure what the heck I was doing.

The longer you're a parent, I believe, the less you feel like you know. I've got a secret. Wait for it . . .

No one does. It's OK.

So if you don't know what you're doing, what do you do? You learn to give yourself grace and realize you're doing the best you can with the tools you've been given. Our tools are often very minimal and, for some of us, nonexistent if we're being perfectly honest.

My toolbox included reading every baby book I could get my hands on. I would figure it out—how to be the perfect mother.

I even minored in human development and family studies in college. I could do this. But surprise—it still didn't come naturally.

Sixteen years in, and I'm realizing the only part that really comes naturally is the love. The rest is dependent on so many other things, like the types of parents you had, how much support you get from your spouse, mental health, and so on. Those are just a tiny fraction of the things that can affect your ability to do the motherhood thing "naturally."

I would guess that almost all mothers love their children. Maybe not upon first sight, but with time and dedication, moms figure it out and bond with their kiddos.

Remember how we're qualifying all the time? "But I love my children!" That's because a mother's love is universal and unconditional.

I believe that sometimes when motherhood doesn't feel natural to me, it is because I need to work on trusting myself and learning to be more confident in my abilities. It may be the same for you.

Thriving in Motherhood Is a Long Game

The love comes naturally, but the rest of parenting takes time, effort, and patience. It's a long game. Not one where we can skip the hard parts and—poof—we are a natural at mothering.

Many of us don't come into our own as mothers until many years into the experience.

That's OK.

We'd never expect our kids to learn how to play the piano "naturally" when no one had shown them where middle C was or where to put their hands.

We can't expect it of ourselves either.

> The love comes naturally, but the rest of parenting takes time, effort, and patience. It's a long game.

Finding a strong support system for the long game is key. This could be family, friends, mom support groups, counselors, and a hobby that only belongs to you.

I know that each situation is different and we've all heard the saying "It takes a village" Well, it does. You don't have to do this alone.

There will be times when you feel like all you can do is survive. But having a support system in place will help. My hope for you is that you begin to have more days when you thrive, more than just survive. Do what you need to do to put that support system together for your mental health and your long game.

CHAPTER 11

Good Moms Never Yell

There is no guilt like the guilt of a mother who has lost her temper. If you've ever screamed at your child while she looked up with fear in her eyes, you know exactly what I'm talking about.

Good mothers don't get angry. They also don't yell. At least that's what I had always believed. There are so many reasons moms can lose control, and it doesn't surprise me with the mental load that we put on ourselves. Again, give yourself grace.

It took me a long time to realize my anxiety manifests as anger. I used to think anxiety was just worry and obsessive thoughts in my head—and yes, it certainly is those things—but it can also manifest as rage. Anxiety makes me a rage monster. I loathe that part of me. I hate admitting it because I feel ashamed.

As a child, I hated that part of my mother. She yelled a lot, and oftentimes I felt fear. My home often felt unpredictable, so I vowed to be different. I vowed to be a mother who didn't yell.

I remember one particularly hard week. I'd had a bad migraine that took me out for an entire day, and the next day I felt angry. By day three of my anger crusade, my anxiety peaked, and I was lashing out at everyone. I hated it, yet I couldn't control it.

When I have one of these angry episodes, for lack of a better term, it feels like absolute chaos in my mind. There is no control, and my anger frequently snowballs to the point where no one wants to be around me. The part that upsets me the most is that I can't predict when my rage will appear. Even the sound of my own children playing in the other room can make me feel like I'm going to lose it. What good mother says that? What mother feels angry when her kid is playing happily in the next room? What kind of mother gets annoyed at the tiniest little thing and yells?

This mom does.

I feel anger, but I feel so much more during these angry episodes.
I feel depressed that the anxiety is back when I had been handling things so well.
I feel hopeless that although I know it will end, it will come back again.
I feel embarrassed I'm sometimes mean to the ones I love most.
I feel like I want to give up.
I feel tired.
I feel overwhelmed by the tiniest thing.

I feel alone. I feel like I'm literally the only one feeling that way in that moment, even though I know I'm not. But anxiety makes me feel like that.

And I hate to say it, but sometimes I feel like I would be better off if I could disappear.

My Anxiety Manifests as Rage and Anger

After an angry fit, I'll have these breakdowns that are as equally ugly. I usually slam things and yell and pick fights with my husband. Then I'll collapse into big heavy sobs in a cycle of self-loathing. It's almost like I finally surrender to the anxiety.

I finally wave the white flag to my family and admit I was wrong. This usually looks like begging for forgiveness from my spouse, and giving hugs and kisses to my kids. Now that my kids are older, I can usually explain the reason for the anger. I say something like, "I'm just really stressed out about how messy the house is," hoping the kids will forgive me.

I feel an immense amount of guilt that those I love are subject to my raging.

It's not pretty to admit you have anger issues. No one wants to admit that. Where's the upside to an angry mom?

As I've started to give myself more grace, I've realized the overwhelming feelings of being a mother are what fuel the anxiety and anger. The anger is a manifestation of the fact that my tank is on empty, no gas station is in sight, and I'm in full-blown panic mode.

It's not that I'm an angry person. Despite feeling inside like that little red fireball from the movie *Inside Out* in those moments, I think I'm more like the character Sadness. Inside, I'm struggling but often too afraid to admit it.

So I let it build and build until, before you know it, I'm breathing fire all over the ones I love while they are looking at me saucer-eyed like, *What just happened?*

We all have our own individual triggers that can send us into a spiral of self-loathing. Maybe you've failed at something that you swore you would never do as a mom. Some cycle you were trying to break in your family or some bad habit you hated about your own mother.

You are infinitely *more* than what is crippling you right now—this cycle that you desperately want to break.

Perhaps it's not so damaging that it's beyond repair? Or, maybe it is. That's why we need a good therapist on speed dial. Am I right?

In all seriousness, though, if anger is a pervasive issue in your home, it might be time to seek help. Anger can be a sign of so many things. For me, it's usually a symptom of my anxiety. For others, it might be from past trauma or from being overwhelmed or from depression.

Anger Is a Healthy Emotion

What if we flip the narrative and tell ourselves good moms *do* get angry from time to time? Maybe even the best moms do. Now, I'm not talking anger like that movie *Mommy Dearest*, where she gets upset about the wire hangers. That kind of anger is traumatic.

Anger is a natural emotion we all feel from time to time. It has a purpose.

Healthy anger is there to warn us when something is off. And maybe a little anger helps your family know you're drowning under the weight of the mother load.

We haven't been told that anger is sometimes healthy and can be good. Instead, we've been told good moms are patient, loving, and kind. They don't damage their kids by *yelling*.

I'm sorry, but I am not June Cleaver.

One night, we were putting the kids to bed, and I had all the windows open. I was giving my kids a semi-loud lecture on listening when I heard the doorbell ring. My first thought was, *Oh crap. What did they just hear?*

The cute older couple at the door had smiles on their faces as I blurted out without thinking, "Did you hear me lecturing my kids?" They smiled like older couples who are done raising their kids do and said, "No. Did they need lecturing?" (I am afraid so.)

I laughed it off while my husband was probably dying to hide somewhere. The kids stood there in their PJs with hair still wet from baths, not knowing what to think.

I realized at that moment this sweet older couple was reassuring me that I'm a great mom. I promise. I just yell a little.

Kids will make you lose it in ways you never imagined

before. And the moms who don't yell (because, yes, they do exist)? Well, I'm convinced they just have a different set of DNA than I do.

I imagine they are horrible at other things, though, like laughing when their kids tell fart jokes or having spontaneous dance parties after dinner (two things I'm great at, by the way).

Kids Test Us in Ways We Never Imagined

While I've made many strides toward ditching my bad habit for good, I'm still human.

I've been known to yell at the three-year-old, "Get buckled, for the love of all things important in this world" so I can finally pull out of the Walmart parking lot, only to look over and see an older lady staring at me. I nod and wave while smiling and saying, "I promise. I'm a great mom."

Because what she didn't see was how he stared into space for a good solid two minutes while I patiently waited for him to turn around and get buckled. And when he did turn around, it was as slow as a sloth with a limp. I'm pretty sure I saw my own life flash before my eyes while waiting. So forgive me for losing it.

To the neighbor who hears me yelling at my kids through our open windows because my children can't tear themselves away from dancing naked in front of a mirror to focus long enough to get not one, but all, of their teeth brushed, I promise—I'm a great mom.

I just yell a little because my kids have the attention spans of woodland creatures with short-term memory loss.

To my friend who watched me yell at the neighbor kids because I caught them putting my child in a trash can, well, that kid deserves my wrath. Besides, I kind of like the neighbor kids being scared of me.

To the random customer service guy on the other end of the phone who hears me yell at my kid to just be quiet before I lose my ever-loving mind, just know—I'm a good mom. It's just they are not used to Mommy having a conversation that doesn't revolve around their egos.

I have to say that I've cut back quite a bit on my yelling. After all, we all need goals for ourselves as mothers, don't we? And not losing my mind is the goal of motherhood—although it might be an unrealistic one, if we're being totally honest.

Yes, we should try to always improve ourselves, but let's not go crazy. We don't need to fill our minds with thoughts of self-loathing if we yell at our kids for breaking a window with a Thomas the Train toy when they are just two years old and so obviously proud of their hard work.

Not that that was my kid.

I'm kidding. It totally was my kid.

Breaking Unhealthy Cycles Takes Time

Breaking cycles takes time and constant effort—and often therapy, a good support system, and potentially medication. Could be all three.

But at least we are in the arena trying to make it happen.

We can combat the feelings of inadequacy by simply owning our own emotions. Try taking your vice or weakness you are struggling with and flip the script:

I yell because I'm overwhelmed, and feeling overwhelmed is normal.
I yell because I'm scared I'm failing at this.
I yell because I'm anxious or depressed.
I yell because I'm tired.

Couple that with past childhood trauma and mental illness like anxiety and depression, and you're bound to feel like a failure before you even get started.

Because having two and three-year-olds will make you yell, right?

And since I'm now entering the teenage years, I can vouch for the fact teenagers will make you yell too.

Breaking patterns and unhealthy cycles is something that takes a lifetime for some of us. Our kids may not think we're perfect, but hopefully they will see we are trying.

Good mothers want what's best for her kids and try their hardest to provide kids with a good environment, and they will also fail.

Good mothers are trying to juggle so many balls, and it's impossible to get it all just right. The best kind of mothers often feel like the worst.

We lose it when we feel like things are out of control. And isn't most of motherhood out of control?

Our Deepest-Rooted Desire Is to Get It Right

We're fighting so dang hard to get it right because that's our deepest-rooted desire as mothers. It's our natural instinct to want to control a home environment where our kids will feel loved, will thrive, and will have every opportunity that maybe we didn't have as kids.

We're comparing ourselves to an impossible standard.

Before you beat yourself up about being too angry or yelling at your kids or whatever other "thing" you're trying to stop as a mom, let me let you in on two little secrets:

1. Your kids will forgive you, and it's vital to ask for that forgiveness. They will respect you more if you can be vulnerable and say you screwed up.
2. Kids are kids. They are unpredictable and certainly not trying to make our lives so out of control. But it's inevitable. Which means a little anger, disappointment, and yelling might happen from time to time. It will be OK.

I promise: if you yell a little, you're still doing a great job. Even if no one on social media admits it, they're probably yelling a little too.

You could google right now, "What makes a good mother?" and find almost two billion different search results. What kind of measuring stick should you be using to find out?

I've got some ideas that will show you that you are maybe already doing it.

Learn to trust yourself.

You know that you have your children's best interests in mind, and you know your child best. All the "experts" out there will try to tell you their own opinion of how to do it, and you ultimately learn to find your inner knowledge. What feels good in your soul as a mom? Do that.

Slow down.

In a society riddled with trying to accomplish tasks, it's often hard to slow down with our kids. I often fall into the trap of being too busy to really see my kids. I find when I slow down and spend time with them, even if it's only fifteen minutes, I recognize I'm doing a good job. I'm trying my best, and my kids love me. Connecting with your kids will fuel the feeling that you are, in fact, getting it right.

> Connecting with your kids will fuel the feeling that you are, in fact, getting it right.

Silence the inner critic.

The voice in my own head is often the worst and most critical one. I can blame society all day long for filling me with feelings of inadequacy, but a lot of those feelings come from my own mind. The lies society tells us often influence our inner voice and affect our mental health. Ideally, we can silence that inner critic and validate ourselves like we would validate a friend. But often we are more forgiving of a friend than we are of ourselves.

While I'm certainly not advocating for yelling at your kids, we can get so swept up in the hopes and expectations we had about parenting that we tell ourselves we're not doing it right when we're really doing just fine. Even if we yell a little.

CHAPTER 12

If You Just Try
Hard Enough

For those of us who don't feel like we slipped into motherhood naturally, my guess is we probably had pretty high expectations. Perhaps we even dared to think we could do it better than our own mothers.

We were going to be different. If we just tried hard enough, this motherhood thing would be fine. We'd be OK. We'd be better than the generation of mothers before us. After all, they didn't know about seat belts and red dye #40, and don't even get me started on the Internet.

We were going to nail it. *Obviously.*

OK, maybe we weren't that overt about it.

Surely I Can Kick This Motherhood Thing in the Butt

I thought that if I tried hard enough, maybe I could do motherhood perfectly. Yes, I know it was a high expectation. I would break old patterns in my own family of origin. I wouldn't have the same struggles as my mother. I guess I had forgotten about the whole part where mental health struggles are hereditary. Instead, I was swept up in this naïve notion I would do it better than most moms before me. That worked great, and I felt like I was totally nailing it until my first child became old enough to stomp her foot at me and say no, or my second came along at full shrieking volume 24-7, kind of sounding like a dolphin *all the time*. I've been screwing up this whole motherhood since then.

In all honesty, I've been a constant disappointment to myself since having my first child.

I know that sounds sad, but I don't see it as sad anymore. I see it as my naïveté as a young woman who thought she had it all figured out.

One of my first low moments as a mom was when my oldest was about two and a half years old. She was the best baby and toddler. The oldest always gets you like that. She got all my attention and was doted on by me and her dad like most firstborn children.

But when I became pregnant with my second, panic set in about having two children. I worried incessantly about my time and love being divided for the rest of her life.

My goal was to get her potty trained before baby number two came along.

I was getting to the point where my belly was getting big, and I *needed* her to figure this out. One particularly hard day, I swatted her on the bum for a potty mistake and put her in time-out, yelling at her. For the record, I never spanked one of my kids again after that.

I immediately went into the other room and sobbed. *What am I doing? I'm screwing it all up. I know better. I am the worst mother. I yelled. Worse, I* spanked *her.*

Recently, I was in therapy, and the shame of that experience came up during a session when I was talking about how I felt like I was failing at something else as a mother. That cute little toddler who was trying so hard to please me, and maybe not quite ready to potty train, is now almost sixteen years old.

My daughter has no memory of it, but here I was working through it almost two decades later. And I didn't even realize that memory was still in there until I did some EMDR (eye movement desensitization and reprocessing) work.

I can look back on that memory now and see the frazzled mom trying so hard and give her grace for her mistake. Everyone had given me the advice to get the first one potty trained before the second one came. I was forcing it. I was trying so hard.

I've finally let go of the shame that I didn't even realize was still hanging out in my psyche, like that annoying neighbor kid who won't go home. The fact that I can even share that story in written form is a testament that I've finally worked through it. It's kind of funny to me now that I sincerely thought if I tried hard enough, I could do everything right and never make a mistake. (Again, with the impossible expectations!)

Recently, I was listening to the podcast *We Can Do Hard Things* by Glennon Doyle. She had Tarana Burke, the bestselling author of *Unbound*, as her guest of the day.

I had an aha moment while listening to Burke talk about her own mother and her failures. She spoke of how she had this moment when she realized her mom desired to love her well, but her failures were due to her own *capacity*.

The idea of desire versus capacity in motherhood was something I had never consciously considered. I knew it in my soul—mothers can only do their best—but I had failed to realize some of us just don't have the capacity for certain things we have the desire for.

Motherhood Is Full of Expectations

We all long to be a certain kind of mother, but do we have the ability to do it based on what we've been given?

Desire to me means love, hope, and longing. Capacity means reality, limits, and abilities. It's OK if our longings don't align with our abilities. Even in motherhood. Most of us have a desire to be a certain kind of mother. Maybe your expectations weren't as unrealistic as mine. I hoped to be the mother who had her crap together all the time.

The cool mom who said yes more than she said no.

The kind of mom who would be totally chill when an entire Costco-sized bag of quinoa ripped apart and went flying all over the kitchen, or when I burned the hard-shell tacos when attempting to make the easiest dinner on the planet.

I expected my own childhood would propel me to do better without many mistakes. I naïvely thought my own trauma would teach me what I didn't want to do and be as a mom (it did), but I thought it would come naturally to do the opposite of the things that I saw growing up. For example, the yelling. I knew I didn't want to yell, but, somehow I still ended up yelling at my kids in the beginning.

I badly wanted to be the laid-back, cool mom. Wasn't wanting it enough? If you just try hard enough and pull up those bootstraps, you should be able to do anything your precious little heart desires. Right?

Now I realize each of us has our own limits and capabilities. Even though the longings of our pre-kid hearts are good and worthy, our capacity to fulfill them is a different story.

Let's discuss further the idea of wanting to be the laid-back mom.

I *literally* cannot be that person all the time. Can I be that person occasionally? Of course.

Some days I don't care about the socks sitting in the middle of the kitchen floor. But other days those same socks will send me into a rage, demanding every happy child content in their own respective rooms must come together in a *Sound of Music* whistle-style lineup and be reprimanded to fix the whole house immediately.

As much as I'd like to be the laid-back mom, I'm just not. It's not in my DNA toolbox. My life experience, my mental illness, and the unpredictability of the kids I am raising all affect the outcome of my day. They have their own unique personalities that I have no control over.

I can only play the role as the laid-back mom as much as I have the capacity to do so. Some days it's easier than others. Some days, not so much.

On the first day of school this year, the first freaking day, I was determined to get all my cherubs out the door with a happy send-off.

At 6:30 a.m. my early bird, who has no problem getting out of bed on time, went to the fridge. He was on top of things. Great. He was dressed and was rummaging around in the fridge for breakfast or to make his lunch.

I was in the other room on the couch trying to rub the sleep from my eyes when I heard a noise all moms dread: a loud crash from the kitchen. I knew it was going to be bad. At 6:30 a.m. on the first day of the school year (it seems important to remind you of that fact), my son spilled an entire vat of spicy Mexican chalupa soup all over my fridge.

It was everywhere.

It was on every level of the fridge.

It was in the grill of the fridge.

It was having a dance party with the dust bunnies *under* the fridge.

It was on the floor and had ricocheted across the kitchen and managed to splatter violently across the cabinets and on the opposite wall too.

Bless his heart, it was also covering his first-day-of-school outfit and soaking his socks.

Y'all. I handled this like a champ. I was sympathetic. I told him it was OK. I reassured him it was no big deal. And I sent him off to go change his clothes while I had to mop my floors and deep-clean the entire fridge, at 6:30 a.m. on the first day of school.

The previous version of me would have lost it. I would have yelled and stormed into my bedroom to wake up my husband to help.

But the parenting gods graced me with patience that day. I was able to calmly ask when he came back into the room after changing his clothes, "Buddy, what happened?"

"I don't know. I was just trying to get some strawberries" was his reply.

My point in telling you this story is not to toot my own horn and show you how I was an amazing mother. It's to point out that some days we just don't know what kind of mother is going to come rolling out of our mouths unexpectedly. Thankfully, that day, I was the laid-back mom.

Tomorrow, who knows.

Our Desires Might Do More Harm than Good

So what is your own capacity? What expectations are you putting on yourself right now that you don't really have control over like you had hoped?

If we outline the wants of our hearts—the things we think we can achieve if we just try hard enough—then we can also check those wants against our innate abilities and talents.

Ask yourself, *Do I have everything I need both externally and within me to achieve the desire of my heart?*

So often, our desire as parents is to make sure our kids have the lives we always longed for as children. Maybe the woman who wants to be the PTA mom always wished her mom didn't have to work full time.

Maybe you want to be the mom who never yells, but your personality is fiery and loud.

Maybe you want to be the crafty, Pinterest mom who makes cute shapes in the Bento lunchboxes, but you don't have a crafty bone in your body.

Maybe you're the disabled or chronically ill mom forcing yourself into being or doing something you're not able to. It would be harmful to you rather than bring you and your children joy.

Those are just a tiny handful of examples of times when our desires don't match our capacity. If we push too hard, trying to achieve these unrealistic expectations of ourselves can lead to resentment, anger, and depression about our roles as mom.

> **Some days we don't know what kind of mother is going to come rolling out of our mouths unexpectedly.**

Our Kids Aren't Looking for a Certain Kind of Mother

Have you ever wondered what your child wants from you? Maybe those wants don't even remotely match up with your own. Maybe your child does not care one bit whether his sandwich is in the shape of a panda. Your child most likely loves your fiery, wild personality.

At some point, we have to kick some of those desires of our heart to the curb, because they are unrealistic or they grew out of something we didn't get as a child.

I know I've been guilty of projecting an ideal onto my children instead of just asking what they want from me. Sometimes parents try to re-create their childhood for their kids in a more idealistic way in order to soothe old childhood wounds. It hasn't been the best way for me to go about mothering. Thank goodness for therapy.

That's what therapy is for, people!

Pursue Growth, not Perfection

With desire and capacity, there's room for improvement. That's the good news. It's not that we should toss aside all the hopes and dreams we had for ourselves as mothers. Growth and improvement will come. We can get there eventually if we work at it and if our goals are realistic, worthy ones.

The vat of soup incident on the first day of school is a perfect example. I always longed to be the mom who reacted naturally to an insane thing my kids did with a calming presence and loving response.

I did it, y'all. I've been practicing patience for sixteen years. A part of me feels like Lizzo: "It's about damn time."

The other part of me knows that growth and improvement don't happen overnight.

Ashley C. Ford, author of *Somebody's Daughter*, said, "You are only good at the things you practice." If you practice something one way your whole life, that's the pattern you stay stuck in.

If you practice something multiple ways, trying new tactics and techniques and methods, eventually you'll find the thing that works for you and your children.

Knowing When to Let Go: The Million-Dollar Question

So, how *do* we determine if we need to try harder or just let go? As with most aspects of motherhood, you have to know what kind of mother load you can handle.

Start by keeping your expectations realistic.
Knowing your capacity is about keeping your expectations realistic, not about giving up on getting better. Yes, try hard, but know when to quit too. You'll know when to quit by how your mental, emotional, and physical health is holding up when you're trying. Does it feel foreign and daunting and overwhelming? Then it might be time to ditch it and reevaluate. Listen to your body.

Trust your gut too.
The way to keep ourselves in check when it comes to desire versus capacity is to trust our gut. One way we can do this is to ask ourselves, *Is this what my kids need, or is this what I needed when I was a kid?* If it feels bad, maybe it's time to ditch it. If it feels like something you might get better at, keep it. Listen to how it makes your mind, heart, and body

feel. If the overall feeling is "I can do this," keep trying. If it feels like it's causing you anguish, ditch it.

Last, figure out what your core values are as a mother.
I've worked on core values a lot in therapy because I struggle with making big (and little) decisions about things. You can apply this to mothering as well. Does it add value to your family's experience, or is it draining everyone and causing discord?

Maybe a core value of yours is to only feed your baby homemade baby food. That's just fine if the process of spending hours making it adds value to your family and to yourself. Some moms really enjoy it.

On the flip side, if you're anything like me, maybe you had no idea how much work was involved in making baby food—so you had to ditch it, because the core value of being a mom who made her own baby food was less important than other things you'd prioritized for yourself and your family. Everyone's priorities are different.

Trying hard is one of those little lies like "wash your face" or "try harder" or "just find the silver lining." All of that sounds good in theory. But if we can slow down and listen to ourselves more, we'll have a better grasp on which goals are worthy and achievable and which pre-kid goals are downright unrealistic.

By letting go of this "just try harder" mentality, I guarantee you'll find out what kind of mother you are and find out what kind of mother your kid needs.

CHAPTER 13

Rub Some Essential
Oils on It

I had a period of my life when I was *really* into essential oils. No, I wasn't pedaling them on the streets or rubbing them on random strangers' foreheads, but I was convinced they were somehow controlling "all the things" in my home.

I thought if I could just rub some peppermint oil on a belly or a forehead that it would control whether a six-year-old spewed the salmon he ate for dinner all over his bedroom floor.

Or I thought if we could just diffuse enough of the right combination of oils in the air, we'd no longer have allergies that have been passed down through generations of noses.

If only you could rub essential oils on a teenager and fix a bad mood.

It was my desire for more control that led me to experimenting with a solution of essential oils to cure all the chaos in our household.

Too many expectations are put on mothers today. I could write a whole book on that alone. I'm here to tell you there is no one way to cure the chaos of the mother load, not even with essential oils.

You can't always cure a baby who is a bad sleeper. Oh, if only there was an oil for that! And don't tell me lavender, because I tried it.

The key to finding healing for whatever is ailing you about motherhood, or the mother load, is finding what works for you and your own kids.

If There Is Anything Constant about Parenting, It's Change

Motherhood is constantly changing and evolving in society and in our homes. Finding a solution or cure to everything that mothering will throw your way is impossible.

For me, homeschooling while working from home during a pandemic, with a husband in health care—really?

So when things are constantly changing and shifting around us, within our parenting journey we have to have coping skills that will help us make it through. To cope during the beginning of quarantine, for example, I implemented a nightly rage walk.

At least that's what I jokingly called it to one of my mom neighbor friends, who I also noticed out walking more than usual. Everything felt unhinged. My routine. My kids. My husband's job. My mental illness. Being quarantined to my house (even for an introvert). Felt. Like. Hell.

So I implemented my nightly rage walk, which was usually after a daily rage cry. The rage walks usually took place about the time my husband came home from the hospital and was able to fully sanitize himself and rejoin our family.

By the time he got home, he knew I was done. Poor guy was juggling working in health care during a pandemic, and I was juggling trying to catapult myself into another dimension to escape reality.

I was going stir crazy and my kids were crying every day. I needed to get out of the house to avoid going completely mad. Things were rough.

My husband could see it in my eyes when I would grit my teeth and say, "I'm going for a walk. Alone.

I walked. And walked. And walked.

I wasn't the only one walking. I saw more neighbors out walking during this time than I even knew existed. *Who are those people?* I had never seen them before, but they lived a few houses down.

Maybe, like me, they were rage walking.

Something that has worked for me to maintain a shred of sanity is exercise. I wish that also meant I had zero problems with my weight (alas, it doesn't). But I have noticed a marked difference in my brain on the days I don't go on a rage walk (or we can just call it a regular walk) versus days that I do.

Walking is my way of coping. If I can just get out and walk, the mother load feels more doable.

Leafy Greens and Yoga, Anyone?

We all have our own ways of coping. Maybe for you it's running or biking. Or maybe you hate exercise (no judgment), and your thing to feel mentally well is all the lights off, some soft music, and some calming lavender oil on your neck.

All of these things help. Do they fix the toddler's tantrums? Of course not. They just help you get through them.

My neighbor's relative would tell you she used CBD oil and her anxiety was gone. Maybe it would work for you, too, or maybe your anxiety would still be there.

My husband thinks all the world's problems can be solved by eating some leafy greens.

My brother has been drilling me constantly that I need to meditate to feel better. Maybe I do. But the one time I tried, it looked something like this:

I sat down, crossed my legs (because isn't that how they do it in the movies?), and closed my eyes.

The words washed over me as I listened to the guide's calming voice. Instead, I found myself wondering:

Am I doing this right?
What does he mean "stop your thoughts"? Who can stop their thoughts? My thoughts are nonstop like a freaking freight train.
OK, concentrate, Meredith. You can do this.
Deeeep breaaath.
In through the nose, out through the mouth. Oh wow, I'm good at this breathing thing.
Oooh. That was a big yawn. Does that mean I'm relaxed? Is the anxiety being released?

Then my brain started in again.

Am I calm enough? What was that noise? OK, forget the noise. Concentrate, Meredith!
Deeeep breaaath.

Yes. I feel it. I'm relaaaaaxed. Aren't I?
This guy must be the most Zen guy on the planet to
make an app. Who decides they are going to be a
meditation guide for a living? I wonder how much
money he makes.

As you can see, I'm still working on the whole meditation thing. Maybe it's not actually my thing. Time will tell.
There *is* value in finding *your* thing and doing motherhood
your way.

Take time to figure out what works for your family, and
then stick to it with confidence. And if one coping strategy
stops working, pivot to a different one.

The Pressures on Moms Today Are a Lot

Because the pressures on moms today are to "get it right" or
rub some oils on it, you'll start to think everyone's opinions
about what's right and wrong when it comes to parenting
matter more than your own.

I don't know about you, but I've heard some opinions
that have made my skin crawl. By the way, your skin crawling is a good indicator it's not for you.

I read a parenting article once that said this:

"WHAT IS WRONG WITH OUR CHILDREN?"
Today's children are being deprived of the funda-
mentals of a healthy childhood, such as:
Emotionally available parents
Clearly defined limits and guidance

Responsibilities
Balanced nutrition and adequate sleep
Movement and outdoors
Creative play, social interaction, opportunities for unstructured times and boredom

OK, so some of those things are realistic when you look at them separately, but if you put them all together and expect they are all going to happen at the same time, it's unrealistic that moms can accomplish all of that.

What about something more extreme, like that kid on TikTok who is two years old, already reading, and can recite all the capitals of every country in the world?

Does that mean every two-year-old should be able to do that?

I'll tell you right now, my two-year-olds barely knew their own names much less the names of every capital city. Could we do more? Of course! Parents could sacrifice their entire lives to their kids. We could drill in those capitals if we really wanted to.

But we already sacrifice so much. We give up our bodies, our careers, our money, our nights out with friends, our sleep, hot food, clean houses, furniture that doesn't have snot wiped on it.

You could give up everything. You'd probably be miserable if you did, but you could.

You could stare into their precious eyes for hours on end, giving them 100 percent undivided attention, and someone would still tell you that it's not enough.

You could donate a kidney, and it wouldn't be enough. You could create sensory bins from Pinterest and crochet all their clothes and grow their food from organic plants in your backyard, and it still wouldn't be enough.

Why do moms believe that they never do enough and everything is their fault? Instead, we should give ourselves grace. We can take the "experts" who tell us what we should be doing with our kids merely as an opinion.

Don't buy into the narrative that this generation of kids is being ruined by me and you and every parent out there trying to raise good humans.

Don't believe the lies that we are ruining our kids because they use cell phones. Yes, they may learn how to say "Alexa" or "Google" or "Siri" very early in life. Don't fret because you text your child from another room in your home. The truth is, texting is a part of our lives now. Like computers, cell phones, and tablets. Can we set limits? Should we set limits?

Of course.

We lose sleep over the demands and pressures we face.

We worry constantly about ruining our kids or screwing them up.

We search for cell phone contracts on Pinterest for our kids to sign saying they'll never take naked photos of themselves if we buy them a cell phone.

We read articles about what is too much and too little screen time and how it's hurting our kids' brains and how it's also great for their brains at the exact same time.

We are trying to keep up with all the pressures, and it often feels like we're just falling short.

How did our parents mentally survive raising kids in the '80s? They let us flop around in the back seat on road trips without seat belts. Helmets weren't required for bike rides. They didn't know where we were for hours. We grew up on Kool-Aid and Fun Dip, for heaven's sake.

Today? So many things are shoved at parents and you can't possibly do it all the "right" way. But I'm here to tell you that you are doing your freaking best. You're trying.

There Is No Right Way Except What Works for Your Family

You don't have to sleep train. There aren't always easy fixes. Essential oils smell nice, but they don't convince a toddler to take a nap.

Don't let society or some article tell you what is wrong with your children or how you're screwing them up. Instead, believe in yourself. Trust that parenting instinct you were given. Because the biggest lie in the world is you aren't doing it right. Have faith you are raising good kids in a new world.

Do what is best for your family.

Your mother load will become lighter if you can ditch the lies society is constantly trying to tell you. But how do you do it when society is constantly in your face?

Put down your phone.
Listen, I don't like this advice any more than you do, because my phone is basically an extension of my hand now. What if we step away from the constant influx of how-to content that has contributed to lies that we tell ourselves? What if we take a moment and focus on what comes from the inside—from our gut, our minds, and our feelings? We're more likely to let go of the noise of what the world tells us parenting should look like.

> **Trust the parenting instinct you were given. Because the biggest lie in the world is you aren't doing it right.**

Practice makes perfect.
With every new stage of parenting, we're still practicing new ways to parent. If it doesn't work out, ditch it. But keep adapting to every new stage and use new methods if something doesn't work. Your goal should be looking for new ways to lighten the load you're carrying.

Nod and smile.
Most people mean well when they're giving you parenting advice. Just nod and smile. Thank them for their idea. It 1,000 percent doesn't mean you have to do it.

Then move forward as you have been and do the thing that is best for your family.

SECTION THREE

Toxic Positivity

"The failure to think positively can weigh on a cancer patient like a second disease."
—**Barbara Ehrenreich**

CHAPTER 14

Just Be Grateful

It was the middle of the pandemic, and I was really struggling with homeschooling my kids.

Let me be clear, I never wanted to homeschool. Never in a million years. It had crossed my mind once or twice that maybe I should homeschool when we ran into hiccups with the traditional school system along the way. My middle child struggled, starting in first grade, with school refusal. Every morning was a battle to get him there and I felt like I was failing him. He eventually grew out of it, thank goodness, because those years made me cry after school drop off and question my parenting abilities on the daily.

But I am also thankful he grew out of that stage because my husband and I were both always joking about how there was no way in hell I was cut out for homeschooling. He gets me.

COVID-19 was like a wake-up call for all of us. Suddenly, freedom was taken away, and many of us felt trapped at home.

We love our little cherubs, but suddenly they were here. All. The. Time.

The announcements trickled in slowly about how we couldn't do things we always had done. First it was restaurants, museums, churches, and concerts closing. I realized this was serious when they canceled the iconic South by Southwest Festival in Austin, Texas.

Then school was canceled for a couple of weeks. Next, state parks, and then the next thing you know you're being judged for taking your kid anywhere public to get some fresh air.

The final gut punch for a lot of people was the announcement that school wasn't going back at all that spring.

There would be no high school graduation for the seniors (including my own niece and nephew that year), and my kids wouldn't get their last year in elementary school and middle school. There were no more school plays, concerts, and carnivals.

And by the way—parents, you get to homeschool now, and your kids can't see their friends.

Good luck.

To say I wasn't adjusting well is an understatement. I started to notice that silver lining trend right away on social media:

Now is the time to organize that closet you've always wanted to!

At least now we can slow down and really enjoy each other!

Do that hobby you've been putting off!

Start a garden!

Here's a fun craft we did with our kids!

Try this science experiment!

I kind of love homeschooling! I get so much one-on-one time with my kids that way.

I was like a deer in the headlights, wondering how to just make it through another day and navigate the seventy-two different apps teachers were using to send us school work in rapid succession.

How exactly was I going to start a garden when I was also trying to homeschool a second grader, fifth grader, and eighth grader? Not to mention I worked from home and had to do things like laundry. To say I was overwhelmed was an understatement. Wasn't my mother load heavy enough already? You want me to add more?

I had *just* gotten my life back after a home remodel, car accident, and severe depression. Now it was ripped away from me again. I could not find the silver lining in all of that. No, thank you.

And if that wasn't bad enough, one day I went online to seek some comfort from a Facebook group I was in. I complained a little bit about the plight of my husband's job in health care, and I got a comment that almost broke me.

At least he has a job.

I immediately felt guilt. She was right. But thanks to the woman's optimistic spin on my husband's job situation, suddenly, my feelings had zero validity. I went from feeling sad to feeling sad, unseen, and unheard, all due to one person's good intentions. But those well-intended words were little more than toxic positivity in a nutshell.

The term *toxic positivity* started making the rounds and

getting more buzz in 2019 when psychotherapist Whitney Goodman (@sitwithwhit) published an interesting list of toxic platitudes and their emotionally healthy alternatives. For example, we can choose to say, "It's pretty normal to have some negativity in this situation" instead of, "Stop being so negative!" Just think about it.

It's like a light bulb went off and people began to realize toxic positivity was making us all depressed. The COVID-19 pandemic shined a glaring light on toxic positivity.

Suddenly, I saw it everywhere. I was angry. Before I was even allowed a moment to have my negative emotion, the toxic positivity mindset propelled me into homeschooling charts, crafts, and baking challenges to make the most of the situation!

I was overwhelmed with thoughts like, *Am I supposed to learn a TikTok dance with my daughter to prove we're having fun during this quarantine?*

"Everyone" was learning a Tik Tok dance or sewing cute masks for people on the front lines or doing art projects.

It felt immediately like I was the only loser in my sweatpants everyday with no makeup on, staring at fifth grade Common Core math, shoving cookies in my mouth, and wanting to cry.

So many of the online posts I read that *did* address difficulties would still tie things up with a neat little bow at the end—a silver freaking lining.

The silver-lining epidemic (that's what I'm now calling it) haunts me. A pandemic does not need a silver lining, thank you very much.

I'd even go as far as to say: this newfound realization that toxic positivity was everywhere lit a fire in me to share the raw, ugly truth about, well, everything.

We cannot always put a positive spin on every situation. This type of positivity is frustrating.

Toxic Positivity Is Dangerous

We stuff our emotions by trying to always remain positive. Some days things don't work out. Sometimes things are incredibly difficult. Life isn't always sunshine and rainbows.

When we stuff down negative feelings by trying to look on the bright side, we don't get a chance to work through those negative feelings. We lose the opportunity to grow.

The amount of parenting books we have today is a perfect example. The expectations are demanding. They all contradict each other, they're confusing, and because of all this conflicting information, we end up just feeling worse about whatever it is that we're doing.

I would even go as far as to say: that toxic positivity culture is exacerbating mental health issues in women.

The mother who is struggling with the load of being a mom is not allowed to speak up and say something, so she's left feeling like she's the only one feeling that way. That's a recipe for depression.

How about the mother who feels so overwhelmed that she wants to run away? Nope. She's not allowed to voice that either. Because people will tell her she's not grateful that she has kids in the first place.

What ends up happening is she stifles those feelings of anxiety until they fester and grow, and maybe something tragic happens as a result.

I know this, because I almost gave up writing completely when someone told me I shouldn't be writing about all the hard stuff.

Toxic Positivity Is Invalidating

Invalidation is harmful to moms because it deprives us of realizing that we have the right to our feelings. What happens next is we feel isolated instead of buoyed by those around us. And isolation leads to fear, depression, and anxiety.

If we didn't suffer from those things already, buying into a culture of toxic positivity will plant those seeds that can lead to mental illness in motherhood.

If we are being told to have "good vibes only!" what happens on a day when we have totally bad vibes? Every mother knows that spending the day with a sick kid or a preschooler who didn't take a nap is one giant bad vibe.

Oh, and what if we show up to a mommy playdate totally rocking the bad vibes? We might feel like we can't open up to our friends about how we are struggling.

When you feel like you can't speak honestly or be vulnerable, that can lead to feelings of depression. Moms need to know they don't have to live in the daily grind alone. They need to know it's OK to have *all* the feels, good or bad or ugly.

Imagine the change we can make in the world by just letting people know they can go through life not being OK. And still be validated in their negative emotions. That's a gift worth giving another person.

Toxic Positivity Is Pervasive in American Culture

Once I started recognizing a positive post or idea that was toxic, whether it was on social media or said to me in real time, I realized that it is pervasive in American culture. We are constantly being told to look for the positive spin—to find the positive and make the best of the negative situation.

Barbara Ehrenreich, author of the book *Bright-Sided*, writes that constant positivity "encourages us to deny reality, submit cheerfully to misfortune, and blame only ourselves for our fate."

When you put it that way, why would we want people to blame themselves and submit to misfortune? We certainly wouldn't want that for our children. Do we want American mothers (or any mother, for that matter) to be wrapped up in blaming themselves for everything bad that happens in their homes?

> Imagine the change we can make in the world by just letting people know they can go through life not being OK.

We Can All Do a Few Things to Combat Toxic Positivity

Try starting here:

Spread solidarity on social media.
I've seen people say how important it is to spread positivity on social media, but what if instead of focusing on being positive, we focus on being in this together? Add comments such as:

> "Me too!"
> "Same!"
> "You're not alone!"
> "That sounds so hard. I'm sorry!"
> "What can I do to help?"
> "I'm here for you."

These are ways we can show other women they aren't isolated in their hard stuff.

Talk about your own hard things.
There is power in sharing your own story. I guarantee you will get negative comments, but I can also promise that if you're going through something hard and you share your story, someone will meet you there. You will find the type of friends who can sit in the yuck with you.

Validate. Validate. Validate.
The worst part about toxic positivity is how it invalidates whatever someone is going through. Validate people by telling them it's not their fault. Let them know you admire

them, and give them a compliment. Really listen and repeat back to them what they're saying.

Encouragement can feel like a lifesaver when you're trying to stay positive during something hard. Telling someone that it could be worse can feel like you've tossed a brick when they are already drowning. By calling out toxic positivity in our culture, my dream is that we as a collective mom community can make a difference in the lives of mothers who are drowning from the mother load.

CHAPTER 15

Negative Nancys

It wouldn't be fair to write about toxic positivity without writing about toxic negativity. No, I don't think this is an actual coined phrase, but it's worth noting there is a reason why people are either half-glass-full people or half-glass-empty people.

Of course, those kinds of people end up marrying each other. Go figure.

Our negative Nancy emotional outlook on life might go unnoticed in our own homes when we're kids. That's most likely because we tend to take on the emotional outlook of those who raised us. In my house, cynicism, sarcasm, and fear often led the way.

I'd like to think these dysfunctional family dynamics bred a good sense of humor. I often deflect with humor and sarcasm when dealing with a negative situation.

So this chapter is for the negative Nancys like myself, because society so often tells us we aren't good because we aren't always positive.

I remember a night when we were driving home from a big family trip. All of us were in the car, it was pitch black, and we were in a hurry to get home. As we weaved our way down the curvy canyon road, suddenly up ahead was a giant elk standing in the middle of the interstate.

Nothing will get your heart pumping like a huge beast who could instantly kill your entire family.

Thankfully, my husband was driving. He slammed on his breaks, the elk darted off, and the crisis was averted. As I tried to calm my racing heart and process out loud what had just happened, I blurted out, "We almost died!" My husband looked at me and rolled his eyes. He looked at the wide-eyed kids in the rearview mirror and said, "We didn't almost die, kids. We're fine."

I was super annoyed.

My racing heart and my life flashing before my eyes (and probably a touch of my anxiety disorder) made me feel like "We almost died!" was a perfectly rational statement.

Obviously, it wasn't. We didn't die. We frankly weren't even close. But my glass-half-empty, emotionally charged, anxiety-ridden self, felt like it for a moment.

It seems silly now, but we got into an argument about it later. I was hurt he made me look crazy and irrational in front of the kids, and he took my statement as possibly scary enough to emotionally scar the kids.

We both had valid points, and we made up and laughed about it later.

My husband is the king of "It's fine," and I'm the queen of "Everything is awful." Sounds like a good balance, right?

When talking about toxic positivity, I can't help but think of all those people who fall into the category of "It's fine!"

You know the ones. Maybe you are one. Which is totally fine. You can't help but lift others up with your bright smile and sunny disposition. You can always give people the benefit of the doubt. You always see the bright side.

I'm not here to criticize those type of people, because frankly, some days I wish I could be that way. I married someone who usually thinks it's all fine.

My point is that my brain went somewhere awful, and his went somewhere calm and serene. I really wish I could take a vacation wherever his mind goes.

The Negative Nancys Come by It Honestly

Were we meant to *always* feel happy? I don't know. I certainly don't always feel happy. If it's a choice, why don't I just choose it? What's stopping me?

Negative Nancys can't easily flip a switch and have the positive attitude. We want to. Trust me, we do. But we are often blocked by past trauma, mental illness, or an Eeyore-like disposition. You know, Eeyore would say, "Wish I could, but I can't." "If it is a good morning, which I doubt." "Days, weeks, months. Who knows?" He cracks me up.

More seriously, Ludwig Wittgenstein, a famous 20th-century philosopher, was miserable all his life. Depressed and anxious, he once wrote in his diary, "There is no happiness for me; no joy ever." Yet minutes before he died, he muttered: "Tell them I've had a wonderful life."[6]

This makes me laugh. Because I'm pretty sure that's what someone will write about me one day. She was totally miserable but also totally content.

A Harvard psychologist named Jerome Kagan researched children and concluded some of them had an easier time biologically being happy, sad, distressed, or moody. He called this propensity for certain emotions to come more easily than others our temperament, and he concluded our temperament is already established in early life.[7]

In my own moments of feeling low, it feels frustrating to think that according to society, I should just *choose* to be happy. I would have chosen that a million times over my struggles with anxiety and depression.

The Idea of Happiness as a Choice Can Feel Toxic

The implication of happiness as a choice perpetuates the stigma that if we aren't thinking positively about life, then it's our own fault. We've discussed in previous chapters how when mothers internalize fault for everything that happens, it only exacerbates their mother load.

Feeling unhappy does not mean you should be ungrateful. It simply means you are struggling through a particular moment or experience, which is part of the human experience.

Happiness Is More Like a Gift, Not a Choice

For negative Nancys, happiness is a beautiful gift, and I'm thankful for it when I can soak it in and really feel it. You are not less-than if you don't have a sunny disposition.

When happiness comes unexpectedly, it feels even sunnier for those of us who don't always look on the bright side. I love laughing at something unexpectedly funny when I've been sobbing about something terrible. Kind of like a crack in a storm cloud.

> Whether you are a Negative Nancy or a Positive Pollyanna, you are important to your kids.

On the days when I can choose happiness, I feel proud of myself. It's like I'm gifting myself happiness.

I would give myself that gift every day if I could.

The important thing to remember is whether you're a negative Nancy mother screaming out, "We almost died!" or a positive Pollyanna making lemonade out of lemons all the time, you are important to your kids.

Both Types of Mothers Are Good

I don't believe that I'm not a good person anymore because some days I just can't see the bright side.

I don't believe I'm weaker than someone else either.

I've done enough therapy to accept my gloomy attitude and feel proud of myself when I feel genuinely happy.

Not all mothers can be put in one of these two camps. That's fine too. The important thing is that we lift each other up and recognize we all have our strengths.

The positive Pollyanna mom could probably use a dose of reality from the negative Nancys of the world. Both should value each other and stop forcing the other to see it their way. So how can we lift each other up?

Value the negative Nancys of the world.
They bring value to the mother load too. They know how to get dirty and bring their fiery attitude to a fight. Don't judge them for being negative or scared of this parenting journey. Appreciate them for keeping your head out of the clouds and helping you fight parenting battles.

Treasure the positive Pollyannas.
If the glass-half-empty gals were running the world, we'd for sure be a swirling Tasmanian devil ball of anxiety. Treasure the Pollyannas who can help us see the good in situations where we can only see the bad. Both kinds of people are very necessary.

And for those of you in the middle, you're the ones who keep us all out of our heads and hearts and help us see the world for what it really is. Not black. Not white. But beautiful shades of gray.

CHAPTER 16

You Don't Have to Smile

I don't know about you, but as I've watched my kids grow up, I'm overwhelmed with a profound love for them I never knew existed before becoming a mom. The whole we-would-die-for-our-kids thing is real, right?

We would do just about anything for them.

We are the cheerleader, the life coach, the shoulder to cry on, the comforter, the nurse, the shuttle bus driver, and the therapist.

Love is wrapped up into everything we do.

It's all-encompassing. The kind of love that forgives quickly. The kind of love that doles out grace in abundance. The kind of love that helps and encourages, empathizes and uplifts. It's unconditional love.

It's the kind of love that would never make us purposely tear our kids down. The kind of love that never ever wants to make a mistake.

It's the kind of love that encourages them to be who they are—flaws and all—and doesn't berate them for being imperfect. It's total acceptance.

Imagine Giving That Same Kind of Love to Yourself

Can you imagine clapping your hands at yourself in the mirror and yelling, "Look at you! You got dressed all by yourself today! So proud of you!"

OK, maybe that sounds totally silly, and it is, but it proves a point: we need to love ourselves unconditionally as well.

What Does Self-Loathing Look Like When You're a Mom?

When I'm having an "I can't" day, it's harder to love myself. Instead, I usually practice self-loathing. I say things to myself like, *Why are you so lazy?* when I go back to bed after the kids leave for school. Or I beat myself up with a thought like, *You could have cooked instead of feeding them take-out again.*

I feel guilty all day long about the should-haves and could-haves of the day.

You could have made something healthier.
You could have read one last story before bed when they asked.
You could have been more patient.

You get the idea. I'm sure you have your own set of special insults you tell yourself.

It takes a conscious, concerted effort to flip that switch from hating ourselves to loving ourselves.

In fact—if I'm being totally honest—I believe that for many of us, women in particular, this is a lifelong battle.

I have a friend who has incredible confidence. We'll call her Sara. Because that's her name.

She's always saying out loud how awesome she is. How smart she is. How clever. It sounds weird, but it's funny, I promise, and it's not in a braggy way. She just exudes confidence I don't have.

Who knows what the heck she thinks or feels on the inside, but I can't help but think that verbalizing self-love helps her more than hiding my self-loathing.

How Do We Pour Love into Ourselves?

We pour love into our kids endlessly, it seems. So where do we start with ourselves? We start by accepting our flaws. For me this has been freeing. It's allowed me to love myself more fully. And a mother who loves herself—flaws and all—will certainly have an abundance of love to pour into those around her.

Next, we treat ourselves like we would our kids. When we screw up, do we berate our children by calling them dumb, stupid, or lazy? Let's hope not. That would be damaging for them (and for us).

Finally, we believe people when they see the good in us. When we get compliments, we say thank you instead of brushing them off as untrue. Why do women do this? It's like when we get a shirt on sale and then feel like we have to confess it was on the clearance rack.

Someone might say, "You're so organized!" to which we respond, "Oh, no, I'm not. I'm a mess. I'm just good at looking like I have things together." Don't do that! Pour love into yourself instead, say thank you.

When we get better at pouring love into ourselves every day despite feeling insecure about our screw-ups, we will become the mothers who pour so much love into their own kids that we will raise up a generation who can't possibly hate themselves.

At least that's the dream. I want to live in a world where our kids love themselves because we loved them well, because we lived the example of what it looks like to love others and ourselves.

> A mother who loves herself—flaws and all—will certainly have an abundance of love to pour into those around her.

When we pour love into ourselves, we also have to take time to be honest about who we are.

Part of Not Loving Ourselves Is About Being Honest

Mothers often feel pressure to put on a happy face. Have you been guilty of this? I know I have. When was the last time you were out running errands with the weight of the mother load on your shoulders, only to be asked how your day was?

I guarantee you, you probably responded much like I do: "Fine." Putting on a happy face, or at least a "fine" face, is what moms do. Even if we don't feel fine at all.

I'm sure if I did my own informal Facebook poll, my mom friends would all raise their collective Internet hands and say they have felt this need to swallow negative feelings as they relate to parenting.

Have we ever stopped to consider that we don't even allow ourselves a chance to *feel* the feelings in the first place because we're so busy trying to hide them?

Mothers are all guilty of going into a closet or the bathroom to ugly cry, working hard to never argue in front of the kids, or trying to always be brave and stalwart instead of scared and fearful.

What if we didn't hide our true emotions or feelings from those around us? Most likely the result would be that we make true, deep, and meaningful connections with others.

If We Love Ourselves, We Feel More Free to Be Ourselves

There will always be people in this world who are uncomfortable with hearing the ugly parts of parenting, mental illness, and life. Without trying to sound superior, I like to think of these people as avoiders. Things that make them uncomfortable are better left unsaid.

Then there are people like me.

I crave emotional connection with other people. I must admit, I've gone out to lunch with a group of women and been frustrated and unfulfilled after leaving the restaurant. Instead of feeling connected to these women I just spent time with, I left feeling more alone than ever, even though I was surrounded by people in the same stage of life.

The reason was simple: because we didn't talk about the hard stuff. We didn't dig deep. We weren't vulnerable enough with each other to make any sort of connection.

Honesty has always fueled connection for me. The times when I have been vulnerable and authentic with others have left me feeling the most connected. Being honest with others makes it harder to lie to myself.

I realize not everyone wants to make deep, meaningful connections every time they interact in public. That would be exhausting, wouldn't it? Can you imagine if someone at Target asked how we were doing and, instead of saying, "Fine," we told the God-honest truth? "I'm feeling really anxious today, and I'm not handling the three-year-old's temper tantrums well at all. I'm thinking of having a drink before noon, and I really, *really* am not looking forward to having sex with my husband when he comes home from work." I believe that person would think twice before asking how a stranger was doing again.

It would be like in that Jim Carey movie *Liar Liar*. We wouldn't be able to help ourselves, and we'd all be slapping our hands over our mouths in shock like, "Make it stop!"

Recently, I went to dinner with my sister. I had to pee

bad as we were leaving the restaurant, but I thought I could hold it until we got home. Word to the wise: if you've had three kids, you can never wait until you get home.

As we left the doors of the restaurant, I pulled a prank on my sister and told her the server was following us because we forgot the to-go box that we purposely left on the table because we didn't like our food. I started to run, and she followed, thinking I was serious.

We got to the car, and I was laughing so hard. She knows I am a horrible liar, so I rarely have successfully pulled a prank on her. But I got her this time.

As we were cry-laughing in the parking lot, the flood gates opened, and I peed all the way down to my ankles. I tried to hop in the car, but we were laughing so hard at the fact I had peed myself that I just kept peeing. It was a puddle, y'all, and I had to sit in it all the way home.

We pulled into my driveway, and I suddenly remembered my cute, hip neighbors next door were having a housewarming party. I knew a lot of the people attending, and they were all standing in the front yard.

I was sitting in my own pee.

I jumped out of the car before any of them could wave me over and ran in the back door. I jumped in the shower and changed my clothes.

I was safe. No one knew except my sister. For some reason, as soon as I got to the party, I confessed to peeing my pants.

Why am I like this? I have no idea.

I kind of secretly wish we would talk about the

embarrassing and hard stuff, because so many women crave talking about the real nitty-gritty of not only parenting but life in general.

So my takeaway is this: let's stop pretending we are one kind of mother and instead pour love into the kind of mother we already are. Let's be more honest with ourselves and with each other. And let's talk more about the times we peed our pants.

CHAPTER 17

People Crave Real

Despite all the perfect-mom Instagram influencer accounts out there with millions of followers, people are craving real life.

And not the people who pretend to be real. Like the moms who are saying, "OMG, my kitchen is such a mess; ignore the background!" while she's making a kale smoothie and her kitchen counters have one cookbook open on them.

People want to see influencers (for lack of a better, less embarrassing term) who *are* real.

That's why I talk about my anxiety and depression and my desire to run away some days.

My posts that get shared the most are the ones that are *raw*. That made me hesitate before I hit publish. That made me wonder if someone I know in real life is going to see them and judge me.

That's why I wrote a funny post about keeping your house clean and poking fun at all those guides we see on Pinterest, and it went viral. Most people don't want another cleaning guide from a mom with white couches and a gigantic, perfectly organized playroom. They want to see mess and clutter and real mom life.

My guide in my first book included getting a dog to clean up crumbs off your floor and soaking dishes in the sink so it looks like you're going to clean them.

Later, of course.

People Want Real, Not Staged and Perfect

Sure, we might enjoy the pretty Instagram pictures for a while, but I guarantee you, we feel less-than afterward. We feel like we aren't measuring up in some way. We put down the phone and look around and wonder what we're doing with our lives.

I followed one such influencer for a long time. She mesmerized me with her long, beautiful hair; adorable kids who always said hilarious things; and her tiny body that fit perfectly into any outfit she was trying to make look messy when really it was perfectly crafted. It felt out of reach, but I kept watching.

Then I opened Instagram one day and up popped a magazine-like picture of an all-white kitchen. The caption read, "Give your counters a facelift with these minimalist items." There were no colors on the countertops. No cups that kids had left out. In fact, there was a pretty pile of neatly stacked mugs, all white, a natural wood-colored cutting board, and a plant in a white vase. It was all just like something out of an HGTV show. None of it felt real.

In my kitchen you'll see a broken cabinet we took the front door off of because the hinge broke and we're waiting on the part. Inside that cabinet for all the world to see are the messy pots and pans I use every day. They are scratched and dented, and not stacked neatly.

I would venture to say my kitchen is more like yours than the one I saw on Instagram.

We stare at screens with people living perfectly staged lives in the little square boxes on our phones we carry around all day. It's the world we live in now. I'm a part of it, and you are too. I feed the machine as much as anyone.

Here's what I hope you will think about as you're sitting among the laundry at the foot of your bed that hasn't been folded even though it's been there a week and you're scrolling through social media.

Are the people you are following on social media helping you feel less alone?

Or do they make you feel *more* alone, as well as inadequate and depressed?

How Do We Become More Real and Vulnerable?

Part of finding vulnerability starts with yourself. Maybe you're trying to curate the perfect Instagram feed or put on a happy face. Or maybe you're trying to curate the ideal version of your life that isn't really you.

If you feel like you're craving more *real* in your life,

perhaps what you need to work on is more vulnerability in three areas.

Being Vulnerable in Friendship.
Are you sharing the most vulnerable parts of you with someone? Because if not, you are probably missing out on finding a true friend.

Do you want someone who will drop everything and come over when your entire family is sick and clean your kitchen? Then you have to be willing to let her in when the house is dirty.

Do you want a friend whose house you can show up at unannounced when you're fighting with your husband? Then you should probably be honest with her about what is going on in your marriage.

You are likely not comfortable getting real with everyone you interact with, so choose one or two people you can trust and start there.

Being Vulnerable with Your Kids.
Are you being real with your kids? Do you share with them your struggles learning how to be a mom? Do you say "I'm sorry"? Saying you're sorry goes a long way with kids; they appreciate it more than you will ever know.

Do you sit in the mess that is life and tell them they have every right to feel the way they do? Can you share the dark parts of yourself when they are old enough to handle it and coach them through overcoming the dark parts of themselves too?

Being Vulnerable with Your Partner.
Are you being real with your partner? Do you let him or her know when you're having doubts about your capabilities? Do you ask for help or share intimate feelings about being afraid of losing the relationship when things get hard? That is one way you can foster authenticity in your marriage.

We Are All Craving Real

In an increasingly virtual world, I crave real life online.

And my guess is there are people out there like me who crave that connection with people who understand the struggles of motherhood.

I'm guilty of staring at my phone instead of connecting with my kiddos or husband. It's a struggle—like, a big one. I'm guilty of saying I'm fine when I'm not. Or telling a little white lie when I can't make it to something because I'm fighting with depression and can't get out of my bed.

I'm guilty of sharing a pretty photo on social media when my hair is really a rat's nest and I'm sitting at home in pajamas that have a hole in them. We're all guilty of avoiding the real, yet we are all craving it.

I want to make a conscious effort to be vulnerable in my relationships both in person and online. I believe it will help me resist the feelings of loneliness and inadequacy. We've all been guilty of faking it. Trying to keep up. Trying to be perfect.

When you can truly be yourself and share with the world that you're struggling and need a friend, that's when the true magic of being real and authentic finally happens.

It's so cliché to say it takes a village, but it does. Maybe the village is in your computer, or is your next-door neighbor, or whoever, but you will only find your village—the true village you crave—by being real.

> **We're all guilty of avoiding the real, yet we are all craving it.**

That I know for sure. So try it. Be vulnerable and say you're struggling, and don't be afraid to ugly cry in front of someone or say, "This is the *real* me."

One afternoon, I ran into a mom friend who also struggles with anxiety disorders. She was on a walk with three kids and a dog, and I was on the way to the store. In our quick interaction before our kids ran into the street, we managed to talk about therapy, meds, and how we both manage anxiety disorder. We talked about the good, bad, and ugly, then we decided to end with a high five. We weren't celebrating; it was just something to let each other know, "I got you, I know you, and I am here for you."

I couldn't help but be grateful as I drove off that I have a few people in my life who I can be 100 percent real with and not sugarcoat a darn thing. That mom has continued to be someone with whom, no matter what kind of day I'm having, I can be real and know I'm not being judged. That kind of friendship is one in a million. But if more of us let our guard down and got real with one another, it wouldn't have to be one in a million.

I know this comes more naturally for some people than others. For me, I've always been emotionally honest. To a fault. I literally don't know any other way to be.

Don't you wish the entire world were like that? "Hi. How are you? Yeah, I'm struggling too." Followed by a hug or high five or whatever. Forget the "I'm fines." I want you to tell me the truth.

Being Real Has Benefits for Parenting

In a 2016 study, it was found that when parents suppressed their negative emotions while parenting, they felt worse about their own well-being, they had a less satisfactory relationship with their kids, and they didn't respond to their kids' needs as well.[8]

That makes me think we can't go wrong by being emotionally honest in front of our kids, as long as the particular issue is healthy to share with the kids.

I'm admittedly an over-sharer. You should have seen how it went when I talked to my oldest about the birds and the bees. "Too much information, Mom!"

Of course, it's a delicate balance while parenting to figure out what your kids can handle, and what's better left unsaid. However, I have found in my own experience that the times when I share with my children honest feelings (even if they're negative ones), the more willing they are to give a hug, encouragement, or even help out.

Let's not dump on our kids and worry them unnecessarily about adult problems, but being open about real feelings can only bring us closer.

Remember, vulnerability fosters connection. If we can talk about the hard stuff in our own homes with our kids, they're more likely to turn to us when their own hard things come up in life.

I'd argue that even your kids crave real. They want honesty when they ask questions, not platitudes. They want openness about hard things. And the beautiful thing is, as they get older, they will likely want to be there for you in your hard times like you've always been there for them. And the only way that comes about is by setting a family dynamic that it's OK to talk about what hurts.

CHAPTER 18

Look on the Bright Side!

Some people slip into the pattern of saying, "Look on the bright side!" or, "It could be worse" because they are genuinely uncomfortable hearing, seeing, or talking about the darkness inside of others.

Mental illness falls into that category because it can be extremely hard to watch someone slip into depression or experience anxiety. As an outsider, you feel helpless. You want to encourage her out of bed with your kind words, but nothing seems to come out right.

Truthfully, we may not want to see strangers fall apart in front of us when we casually ask, "How are you?" because if they did, we'd have to stop whatever it is we were doing and address their pain. It would be cold and inhumane to ignore that.

That's a lot of responsibility, right? It takes time and effort to show empathy. And what if we're on our way to work and running late and someone tells us she's falling apart? It's hard to stop what we are doing and be in that moment with her.

When we see another human suffering, we want that

suffering to go away so we can go back to our own happy place. As harsh as that sounds, we're all guilty of it.

Watching someone fumble through motherhood is no exception.

Have you watched a friend walk through a hard parenting stage and you wanted so badly to tell him how to do it better? Have you watched a friend suffer through infertility and felt guilty because it is easy for you to have kids? Have you struggled to watch a new mom figure out how to breastfeed, and you wanted to whip out a boob and do it for her?

It's human nature to not enjoy watching someone struggle. It's hard to watch.

That's what makes opening up and being vulnerable so freaking hard. We fear rejection. We fear someone looking the other way. We fear whispers about us. We fear others not thinking we are good mothers. We fear others will believe we can't accomplish great things because we struggle.

It's a lot to digest. And isn't it funny how one negative comment or one person saying, "Look on the bright side" can be the one thing that you hold on to when it may be unattainable?

We Need to Be Able to Talk About What Hurts Anyway

It can feel hard to look on the bright side when we're really struggling. A few years ago, I had an experience that changed my life. I come back to it often when I sit down to write something that is scary to me.

I just had my third baby and was no stranger to post-partum depression. I lived far away from my family and didn't have much support. With two toddlers at home, to say I was on the struggle bus was putting it lightly.

I was in a bad place. No one was holding the baby for me while I napped. No one was bringing meals. No one was offering to fold laundry while I nursed around the clock.

And I'll just throw in there: my youngest also had severe colic and food allergies and woke up every hour and a half to nurse. I was a *mess*. A hot, sticky, sleep-deprived, angry, annoyed, frustrated, depressed, anxious mess of a human being.

There are not enough adjectives to describe how big of a mess I was. I was in the trenches of young motherhood, but I was in the trenches of depression too. My blog became my outlet. I put it all out there. I put out there the negative thoughts, the depression, the anxiety, the OCD, the frustration with no sleep.

The experience of feeling alone and having no help was eating me alive. I needed to write about it and reach out to other mamas who had been there.

I needed to write about it to also help other mamas feel less alone in their own struggles.

I needed to speak about my hard things to let them go.

My saving grace was typing it away on my computer and sending it out to the universe. It was cathartic to me—an emotionally honest, brutally authentic person—to put it out there, to release the feelings and be free of all of them.

But a few weeks into all that venting and releasing and feeling free, it came to my attention that some of my family members were reading my blog and were worried about me. They were talking about me.

I was confused. Why was no one talking *to* me if they were worried? Why were they talking to each other instead of reaching out to help? I felt like maybe I should just be silent instead. I felt completely and utterly judged, but worse than that, my outlet for releasing all the negative heartache of a difficult time in my life became tainted. Writing felt ruined. I felt as if being honest and vulnerable had backfired, as if I would never write another word again.

Yes, I have a flair for the dramatic.

My blog had become my safe space to vent, commiserate, and felt like I had a whole community of mamas behind me cheering me on. I guess I needed that when I felt alone in real life.

Bless my sweet husband during this time. If it weren't for him telling me to not give up writing, I would have stopped right then and there.

Looking back, I'm grateful for the experience because I learned more about myself than if that had never happened. I learned that my voice in that space was important even if it made other people feel uncomfortable. I learned to forgive. I learned to speak up without shame. And I learned that some people will never be OK with talking about the ugly parts of life.

Talking about the hard stuff is how we can help others feel less alone. If you talk about what hurts and avoid feeling like you always need to be looking on the bright side, you'll find your people.

You Have to Find Your People to Sit with You in the Darkness

The people who are not comfortable sharing in your ugly and sticking with you as a friend during the difficult times are not your people. We need friends who will not force us into looking on the bright side, but instead sit with us patiently while we get there on our own.

Your people are the ones who reach out to you during the darker times. Your people are the ones who won't try to tell you it could be worse.

> **Talking about the hard stuff is how we can help others feel less alone.**

When people feel compelled to tell you to look on the bright side, it's often because they just don't know what else to say. We are all guilty of diminishing someone else's suffering because of our own need to look away or because we don't understand it. Instead, extend grace. That does not mean you should stop sharing who *you* are. It just might mean you haven't found your people yet.

How Can We Foster a Community of Like-Minded Friends?

Chances are, you're now going to see examples of toxic positivity everywhere. Does that mean we toss aside those friends who continue to do this to us?

I don't think so. Instead, rooting out these sometimes-hurtful things people say to us in our darkest hours takes bravery and work.

How do we do it?

Gently lead by example.
An example is the greatest teacher. Have you known someone who just exudes empathy and understanding? I have.

I'm usually drawn to that person and watch how she interacts with others so that I can learn to be a better friend. If we can start taking the overly positive phrases out of our own vernacular and replace them with empathetic phrases, other people will notice and follow suit.

Speak up and let others know they invalidated your feelings.
Speaking up feels hard because it requires bravery and puts us at risk for confrontation with those who can't handle the criticism. I know. I've been there. If someone doesn't feel like a safe person to be open and honest with, that's OK. She isn't one of your people. For those who just need a gentle reminder, you are helping them be a better friend. I think being gentle is key, because they likely never meant to invalidate or hurt your feelings.

Try not to take it personally.
As a highly sensitive person, this one is hard for me. I take the whole world personally. It's especially hard when you're the one suffering already. But part of learning to do this is through pouring love into ourselves and being confident in who we are. The more we can practice self-love and confidence, the less the toxic positivity will affect us.

SECTION FOUR

Mental Illness

"If you can't fly, run. If you can't run, walk. If you can't walk, crawl, but by all means, keep moving." **—Martin Luther King Jr.**

CHAPTER 19

We Don't Talk
About That

I wish mental health would not have been such a taboo subject when I was growing up in the '80s and '90s. People didn't talk about anxiety and depression. At least not that I remember.

I have vague memories of a wide array of mental health issues running through my family. I just didn't have the verbiage for it. No one was saying words like *depression* or *anxiety* around me. I learned to draw my own conclusions.

My maternal grandfather was an abusive alcoholic. My early memories of my mom talking about her childhood are fuzzy, but she made lots of comparisons between how hard she had it versus how hard we had it as kids.

So I knew things were rough for her. I knew I had cousins who struggled with addiction, depression, and anxiety. I knew my own mother struggled with something—bipolar disorder or something like that.

We knew things were different with some of these family members, but we didn't talk about the actual root of the behaviors and addictions.

I also remember recognizing the stigma. I knew family members who were medicated, but we didn't talk about it.

No one sat down with us as kids to explain why things were volatile in our home, when my friends' homes were peaceful. No one apologized for the blow-ups and fights fueled by mental illness. No one explained the *why* behind it all. At least not that I can remember.

Our family seemed to be in continuous turmoil and survival mode. Looking back, there were definite signs I was struggling with mental health in childhood. I was always labeled as the worrier (true) and the whiner (also true) in my family. I lived in a constant state of what-ifs and stress. I crawled into my parents' bed often, frequently waking in the middle of the night and telling them I had a bad dream, even when I didn't. My mind would often race with fear and worry. I felt unsafe a lot of the time.

One of my earliest memories of a breakdown or panic attack was in fifth grade when I was ten years old. I had read a book called *Night of the Twisters*. Do not recommend it. Zero stars. I don't know why any child—much less a child prone to worry—would ever want to read this book. But I was an avid reader. Maybe it was for a school book report. Who really knows.

After I finished that book I was convinced we were going to have a tornado. That night. At my house. I vividly remember having a complete and total meltdown. My parents had gone to bed and locked their bedroom door because parents of the '80s did that sort of thing, but I was insistent someone take me seriously.

My sense of panic was escalating quickly, and I broke down into body-wracking sobs outside their bedroom door. I wanted them to let me in because, in my mind, we were in imminent danger of a tornado. I laid in the hallway kicking their door in protest.

This went on for what felt like hours, with me in hysterics, until my older brother finally stepped in and dragged me to the front door. He swung it open to reveal the starry, clear night sky. He said something to the degree of, "Look, Meredith! There is not a cloud in the sky. There is not going to be a tornado!"

After that, I was satisfied enough to calm down.

Throughout childhood, scenarios like this played out often. Me being irrational. Being told by my parents I was being dramatic. Me crying, worrying, and begging for someone to take me seriously about all the worry, fear, and stress going on in my little brain.

It could involve anything. My common triggers were worries about being late to places and about whether our doors were locked.

I would get up in the middle of the night and check doors, and I'd frequently lose it when I knew I would be late to school. I worried about my parents' money problems and did not sleep well.

My family was full of dysfunction and unhealthy dynamics, but as a kid I didn't have the skill set to recognize that, and my parents' generation didn't have the skill set to talk about it.

Nothing was done when I was a kid. I didn't go to therapy. There were no loving sit-downs trying to get to the root of my irrational fears. There wasn't a lot of empathy when I was freaking out about being late to school or church or work.

One valuable lesson I learned from my childhood is to sit down with my kids and talk honestly about their fears and stressors.

I cried a lot and worried a ton, but for the most part, I was a compliant, well-behaved kid with good grades and lots of friends, who otherwise had a happy childhood.

Do I wish I would have gotten the skills and tools I needed to cope with stress earlier in my life? Of course. One valuable lesson I learned from my childhood is to sit down with my kids and talk honestly about their fears and stressors. Let them pour their hearts out and empathize with them. I want to really listen and let them know they are validated and safe.

Anxiety and Depression Are Usually a Lifelong Battle

I haven't always fought my battles with anxiety and depression gracefully.

I've experienced depression after break-ups and panic attacks, to   mood swings, terrible, irrational fights, and skewed thinking as a newlywed while taking birth control. Not to mention postpartum depression and anxiety that started with my first child.

Despite all those warning signs and knowing my family history, it took me years to ask for help and then accept it from both professionals and people in my life.

I don't dwell on the fact that I needed help when I was a child and didn't get it. But I share in the hopes of letting others know how anxiety and depression can manifest in a child. I wish someone had paid more attention, but I'm also aware that the stigma around these issues was prevalent at the time.

Recognizing and Talking About Mental Illness

How do we start the conversation about something that others might view as awkward, too personal, and vulnerable?

First, educate yourself.
I always had a fascination with mental illness and ended up getting a degree in psychology. I loved studying the brain and why people act the way they do. I loved analyzing people's behavior.

Even with class after class about the brain and behavior, I still found it difficult to apply the knowledge to myself. I never went to college to diagnose myself. Who wants to do that? I went to better understand the world around me.

And I did. There was still something that kept me from applying what I learned to my own issues.

It wasn't until I started therapy years later that I took some of the things I already knew about the brain and behavior and started applying it to my *own* brain and behavior.

In therapy, someone walked alongside me, saying, "This is why you are like this, and hey, it's OK. It's who you are. Here are some tools to help you."

When my therapist would speak on some of the subjects I had previously learned in school, it was like hearing it all for the first time because I was now applying it to myself.

If you're suspicious you have an anxiety disorder or depression, speak with a professional about it. Read a book on the topic. Even do a deep dive into anxiety on TikTok if you have to.

I'm not recommending you seek treatment for your mental illness from TikTok—because, let's be honest, some people over there are doing some weird things. But rather, learning about it can only help you further recognize and seek out the real, professional help you need.

So often as mothers, we put our own needs to the side, but when it comes to depression, anxiety, or any mental illness, it's vital you take the time to learn about it so you can seek the help you may need.

Second, accept yourself
Sounds like common sense. We should all be able to accept ourselves, right? But do we accept ourselves enough to forgive when we do something because of our mental illness? Not usually. Usually, we are ashamed. We loathe the part

of us that needs medication or thinks about never waking up again.

Do we accept our mental illness enough to work daily to fight negative thoughts and feelings about it? Do we accept who we are? Mental illness and all?

Sometimes I watch reality TV and see people who seem to have an overabundance of confidence and an "I don't care" attitude. I get jealous. *Where did all that confidence come from?* That's why I like reality TV so much. It's like a train wreck of overconfident people who are so different from me that I can hardly fathom it. And I can't look away.

Tell someone off? No problem. Wear something crazy and not care? Sounds good.

Parent your child by giving her Mountain Dew before her Little Miss America performance at the age of six? No worries.

Go on a dating show and tell the whole world that you *know* this guy is meant for you even though it's been three days and he's dating twenty-five other girls at the same time? I got this.

Some people are just born with that confidence. I wish I was, but I am more like the phobia person. Even if that means we tell someone, "Hey, so I have this major fear around vomiting because of my anxiety disorder, and if your kid pukes, just know I still love you, but I'm probably not going to hang out for a week or so."

Once we learn more about how depression and anxiety can be out of our control, it's easier to accept. Part of accepting mental illness will lead you to seek out treatment for it. Remember, we already know how to pour love into ourselves, so if we practice self-love and accept our mental illness, we're going to seek the help we need.

Third, seek help.
I will never forget the first time I went to a practitioner to get some medication and the shame I felt admitting I wasn't handling my anxiety how I wanted to. I was so grateful for a kind and gentle doctor who reassured me it was OK not to be OK. It wasn't a failure. But in my eyes at the time, I was in such a low place, I did feel like I was a failure.

That doctor helped me get the treatment I needed and helped me to accept myself, flaws and all. If he hadn't been as gentle and kind as he was, I might have left there still unmedicated and hopeless.

Instead, I learned to accept I was struggling and got the help I so desperately needed.

By Seeking Help, We Help Others Hold Us Accountable

Seeking help is the first scary step. Whether it be meds, self-care, or talking to a therapist (and it's totally OK if it's all three), seeking help will be the fastest way to teach yourself how to talk about mental illness.

While we've talked a lot about being open and honest, we haven't talked as much about why it's important to be open and honest about mental illness too. For me, it's about others helping us be accountable. When you tell a doctor, a

friend, or a family member about your mental illness, suddenly you're not going through this all alone. If someone is
on your side and advocating for you, he or she will gently
help you stay accountable. This is why people get running
partners or diet buddies. Even superheroes have sidekicks.
We often need people to be our cheerleaders in life. Whether
it's a doctor prescribing meds, a therapist making you do
your therapy homework, or a spouse making sure you get
out of bed every day, having an advocate can help us start
to normalize what's going on within us.

Though we didn't talk about depression and anxiety in
the '80s, a shift is happening and it's one that I'm so grateful
for. The more specific topic of motherhood and mental illness is one I hope to normalize through these pages.

For many of us mothers, it feels shameful that we are
trying to raise humans while mentally ill. But part of the
mother load is about mental illness, because so many of us
are struggling with it. It's time we get more open and start
exploring what that means for us and our children.

CHAPTER 20

When You Can't
Walk It Off

Years ago I vividly remember sitting on the edge of my bed sobbing to my husband, "I feel so broken." I was knee deep in potty training and babies, and my relationships were suffering because I did not have a strong grip on my emotional outbursts and my mental health.

I had yet to figure out the magic combination of medication, therapy, and self-care needed to help me cope with my anxiety and depression, and I felt hopeless. The story I was telling myself about my own mental illness wasn't helping me get through that difficult time. I was telling myself that broken things shatter. Broken things aren't reparable.

Broken things can infect everything else around them.

It's like those four eggs in my fridge. Only one had a crack in it, but it leaked its egg guts all over the other eggs in the container. When I went to get just one egg out of my fridge, it had this thick, solidified yellow yolk goo on it from the cracked one that had already been tossed. Even hot water couldn't get rid of the goo. So at a certain point, I said, "Screw it" and threw four perfectly good, although goo-covered, eggs away. What if that happens to people? What if I am broken and I break and leak onto those around me? I know that is not how it really works because our brokenness surely isn't contagious.

I Am Not a Mistake

I used to think that nothing came into this world already broken. Humans certainly don't. Have you met a baby? Or a puppy? They are perfect.

It's a radical thought, the notion that I'm a whole person, even with a mental illness. I used to think maybe after this life, in heaven, I'd be something different and my mental illness wouldn't be a part of me. It's fine if I'm miserable now, because one day all the brokenness is going to disappear—poof! You're a spirit now, but surprise, your brain finally works.

I didn't want the mental illness to exist at all. So instead of accepting it, I labeled it as something broken. I didn't see myself as a whole person. Instead, I imagined myself like a puzzle missing one piece. It's infuriating to get to the end of the puzzle and not have all the pieces, but there's not much you can do about it because someone probably sucked it up in the vacuum. Right? Regardless, it felt like a piece of me was missing. But I am not a mistake, even though I felt like I was.

My favorite cliché when thinking about my mental illness is, "God doesn't make mistakes." Then I digress and think, *Excuse me, have you seen some of the weird things that exist? Like flying cockroaches? If He doesn't make mistakes,*

He has a sick sense of humor to make a Texas-sized cockroach that's unafraid of humans, that can fly.

Many times, I have thought that when God made me I was a big ole fat mistake. Some wires got crossed in my brain, or a part of me was forgotten on the assembly line. (Raw, truth, right?) Maybe He muttered, "It's fine. She is deathly afraid of germs, heights, and anything unpredictable, but it will all work out." God must not have realized it would only all work out fine until motherhood happened. Then those pesky little wires would get crossed and short-circuit.

If you have tried to parent while depressed or anxious or with obsessive compulsive disorder, you know what I mean. Have you seen that fun game babies like to play where they throw their pacifier, food, or sippy cup down on the floor 847 times so you will pick it up for them over and over and over? First, I have to ask: why do we keep playing that game? Second, that crap gets old real fast when you're already strung out on lack of sleep and depressive thoughts. No wonder moms feel like they are going to lose their crap.

It was a journey for me to realize and accept that I needed help. Talking with a doctor who prescribed the right meds and then going to counseling helped me realize that I am a whole person. I am not a mistake; everyone has their struggles, and this is mine.

What Are Anxiety and Depression?

Through a quick google search it's apparent that depression and anxiety are legit illnesses. Imagine that! We all go through periods of anxiety and depression in our lives because that's part of the human experience, but clinically diagnosed anxiety and depression are different. I've wondered if we polled the entire human race with some big, gigantic touchscreen in the sky, if we would all answer that yes, we are either (A) Depressed, (B) Anxious, or (C) Both.

Show me a mom or dad who isn't anxious at some point in their parenting journey. Show me a parent who hasn't been depressed because of a situation or circumstance.

But pervasive depression and anxiety aren't situational or due to temporary circumstances; they are illnesses of the mind.

According to the Centers for Disease Control and Prevention (CDC), the symptoms of depression look similar to this:

Someone who is depressed has feelings of sadness or anxiety that last for weeks at a time. He or she may also experience—

- Feelings of hopelessness and/or pessimism
- Feelings of guilt, worthlessness and/or helplessness
- Irritability, restlessness
- Loss of interest in activities or hobbies once pleasurable
- Fatigue and decreased energy
- Difficulty concentrating, remembering details, and making decisions
- Insomnia, early-morning wakefulness, or excessive sleeping

- Overeating or appetite loss
- Thoughts of suicide, suicide attempts
- Persistent aches or pains, headaches, cramps, or digestive problems that do not get better, even with treatment

Anxiety and depression are often grouped together like the less desirable form of something delicious such as peanut butter and chocolate.

They get grouped together because they have overlapping symptoms (like anger), and many times, the anxiety and depression like to fight over which one gets to take over your brain that day and cause havoc.

When the symptoms of anxiety or depression last a long time, often we can feel intense, uncontrollable feelings. Some of those include fear, panic, worry, and the inability to get out of bed and parent.

I imagine if you're still here and reading, you've felt some of these feelings and have wondered how you were going to do the whole motherhood thing when you feel like that leaking egg in my fridge oozing your pain and suffering all over everybody in the house.

When I first had a panic attack in college, I experienced shortness of breath, rapid heartbeat, and feeling like I was going to die. I just waited it out in my little room in my apartment, and no one needed to know about it. No one did for many years. I was able to mostly continue with normal life once it was over.

It wasn't until I became a mother that I was keenly

aware I had a problem that needed additional help and resources, because if you're having a panic attack while driving your kid to preschool, that could be problematic.

When you're in charge of other humans, you can't always just ride it out in the quiet of your bedroom with the door shut.

Imagine trying to take deep breaths through a panic attack with a toddler on the other side of the door yelling, "Mooooooommmyyyyy, I need you to wipe my butt."

When We Are Mothers, It's Hard to Normalize Mental Illness

Because we are so wrapped up in the lives of tiny dictators (aka children) who demand so much of our attention, we often forget that depression and anxiety are real illnesses that need professional help much like heart disease.

If you're suffering from undiagnosed mental illness, you will most likely need additional help as a mama even if all your life you've been managing just fine.

When I was a younger mom of two littles, I got hyper-focused on one of my kids' bowel movements. Not one of the BMs, but *all* of them. As one does. This is totally normal for moms. We talk about poop like we talk about the weather. "Did you see that diaper last night? I was totally gagging. I had to take it straight outside to the trash because it was so foul I thought it might resurrect a demon or something."

When my son was a baby, he had some gastrointestinal

issues that turned out to be related to food allergies. I could often find myself poking around in his poo (I'm sorry if you're now gagging) to see if there was any blood in it, because he had a rare allergy disease as an infant called FPIES (food protein-induced enterocolitis syndrome), which caused his GI tract to bleed, and blood would appear in his poop. Super sad, but it was easily fixed by some dietary changes of mine. Because I was breastfeeding, I had to cut out dairy and soy.

Just kidding, it wasn't easy. It was the longest fourteen months of my life to go without cheese, because . . . *cheese*.

I became kind of obsessed with this kid's poop and gas issues and all things GI-related. I became fixated on how much he ate and what I ate and whether a Ritz cracker I was craving had a tiny bit of soy lecithin in it.

It was a dark time. Because also . . . no cheese.

During this time I was also suffering from postpartum depression and anxiety that was untreated. Let's not even mention the fact I was also diagnosed several years later with OCD, hence the obsession with his poop consistency. I was focused so hard on my kid's bowels, I was forgetting to pay attention to my mental health. Finally, during that year I had a breakdown, I guess, because I went to that compassionate doctor and got on some medication.

Struggling with mental illness while you are a mother is no easy task.

196

My hope is that through these next chapters, you can find yourself in the pages if you struggle, and you can seek the professional help you need. Because struggling with mental illness while you are a mother is no easy task. It requires forgiveness, courage, and strength beyond measure.

It requires turning inward when your focus is elsewhere. Like on the poop.

You are not broken because you struggle with depression and anxiety. You just need a little extra love, help, validation, and encouragement.

CHAPTER 21

Depression Is a Beast

I remember one particularly bad weekend when I broke down because my depression was confusing even to me. I wanted to do something fun as a family. I even suggested it. Yet the morning of, I was angry—lashing out at everyone and super annoyed by the whole ordeal of getting ready to go. My husband finally stopped me mid-tirade and asked,

"Do you want to go?"

"Yes!" I barked back.

"Well, then, why don't you change your attitude about going?" he said calmly.

Oof. That hurt.

He was 100 percent right. My attitude was sucking royally. I went into my room and shut the door and sobbed. I cried because I realized one part of me wanted to go, but my depression was sending me a different message. Another part of me wanted to eat chips in bed while watching murder shows in a quiet house. I wanted to lie in bed for hours or maybe even days.

I mean, most moms want to do that, am I right? We are a tired crew in general.

Depression makes me need sleep. Crave it. And yet I don't enjoy the time in bed. Instead, I use the time to become my own personal punching bag.

You suck because you planned this fun outing and now you're acting like you don't want to go. PUNCH!

You aren't a fun mom. PUNCH!

You're better off without kids. PUNCH, PUNCH!

It's not an enjoyable experience to lie in bed all day punching yourself (figuratively) for being depressed. I know. Because I've done it.

My depression confuses me because it's something I haven't dealt with it as much in my life. Anxiety? Yes. OCD? Yes.

But the depression part I'm still figuring out.

Depression Is Its Own Unique Beast

I have newfound empathy for those who struggle with deep, dark, debilitating depression.

I remember an incident where my two-year-old was struggling with a limited vocabulary. We were both struggling, let's be honest. He woke up one morning and seemed frustrated before the day even began. By 8:30 a.m. it felt like I had lived a lifetime, died, and come back to life as a ghostly, less patient version of myself.

I was irritated as I put oatmeal in front of him. I didn't understand what he was requesting for breakfast, so I figured brown sugar oatmeal (a fair-weather favorite) was good enough. As I set the breakfast in front of him, I tried to understand why he was frustrated. Did he really want a waffle? I couldn't figure it out.

So I asked him, "Waffle or oatmeal?" in an effort to have him articulate what he needed. He muttered, "Meal." But as he looked at his "meal" sadly, he took a tiny bite and kept crying. He started to say, "Mommy" over and over. He could only say "Mommy," even though I knew he needed something more. Maybe it wasn't about the oatmeal at all. I just remember he was frustrated, and so was I.

That's often how depression can feel—like wanting a waffle but not being able to articulate you want a waffle because you're a two-year-old, and "waffle" is hard to say. So you say something you don't mean, like "meal." Then you get the oatmeal from someone who loves you and wants to make you happy, and you just cry through the entire bowl of oatmeal.

Depression feels confusing to me that way because I want to do the things I love, but depression stops me from doing them. Talk about a confusing battle to have with yourself daily.

Depression looks like wanting to run a marathon but just not being able to because you're injured. Except the injury isn't something obvious like a break. It's something invisible like a muscle tear. It looks like wanting to spend time as a family but not being able to because you want to be alone.

It looks like wanting to work out, write, draw, or do

whatever it is you love to do, but not being able to because your mind is asking you, "What's the point?"

I tried to explain all of this to my husband later that evening after our argument.

I apologized and cried and said, "It's the worst feeling in the world. I don't know how to explain it."

I want to be happy, but I'm not able to find joy. It's a confusing, frustrating feeling. But most of all, it feels like disappointing yourself and everyone around you every day.

Those are some dark thoughts to have on days when you're already not feeling like the best human in the world. Mothers want so badly to be the supermom, but instead, often we're dragging ourselves through the day for the sake of our kids.

It's been a long process to realize these bouts of depression come and go, and I just have to drag myself through them like you're dragging a tired toddler who's just had too much fun at the zoo, doesn't want to leave, but also doesn't want to walk to the car.

I had a temporary stint with postpartum depression after my first baby, and a very short battle with situational depression after a bad break-up from a loser ex-boyfriend in college. The first time I recognized that it was affecting my daily life was when my youngest started full-time school in first grade. The anxiety I was used to. I had lived with it my whole life. But this? This was a whole new experience for me.

I was suddenly blindsided by the fact that some days I felt so heavy and like I just couldn't face the day even when there were a million things to do. Frankly, I just felt tired and sad a lot. It's not out of the norm for someone like me with mental illness to experience depression too. But I guess I wasn't expecting it. I never do on the days when I can feel it.

One night when I was feeling particularly low, I sat on the couch listening to the baby of my family, who wasn't really a baby anymore, read this book all by himself. Then it hit me why I might be struggling. It's because my littles are now big. Suddenly, I was enjoying running errands without kids in tow and looking forward to silence. But there was also this palpable taste of the emptiness that is coming my way rather quickly as my kids grow up. As a young mom it was particularly hard to hear that it goes so fast. I probably rolled my eyes too. But now I'm mad they were right.

I miss so many things about those early years. I know I enjoyed it as much as I possibly could. I lived it. But a part of me is seeing the house one day that will be permanently empty, and it's coming at me fast. And I find myself catching my breath at simple moments like my youngest reading a book by himself. I found myself trying to memorize the sound of his voice and the twinkle in his eyes when he got to a silly part.

I've always known motherhood is heartbreaking work, but I just didn't expect for it to feel so *heavy*. And it felt heavy at that moment. Motherhood is soul-crushing work while also being soul-filling. Perhaps it's even devastating some days while simultaneously being full of joy.

It was hurting me to watch my kids grow up so quickly,

and it was bringing up all my deepest fears. So much of my life had been wrapped up in theirs, it felt like my heart was breaking. I slipped into a depression.

For months, I kept telling my husband I was in a funk. I eventually figured out it was worse than just a funk when I didn't want to leave my bed every day. But when you're a mom, you get out of bed and keep doing it, even though it feels like twenty-pound bags of flour are strapped to each leg, making you sluggish and tired. You push through.

> Motherhood is soul-crushing work while also being soul-filling.

Thankfully, I went back to my doctor, and he switched my meds. It was life changing for me, and maybe even life saving for this stay-at-home mom. I am fortunate to be able to stay home with my kids, but it's not roses every day, and it's not for everyone. There are days I love it and days I, well, want to stay in bed.

Depression for Stay-at-Home Moms Seems Particularly Hard

Please don't think for one second that I don't believe working moms work hard—I am a working mom. But when I was not working outside of motherhood, my depression was so much worse than when I was working in a job, so I am only speaking from my own experience and that of other stay-at-home moms I know.

It boils down to one key aspect of being a stay-at-home mom: not much outside validation. Stay-at-home moms know they are contributing to society, because, duh. But nobody is running around high-fiving stay-at-home moms for wiping the kitchen counter for the eighty-seventh time that day. Kids aren't coming home from school and saying, "Good job, Mom! You finally remembered to switch the laundry that's been sitting in the washing machine for four days." Partners aren't always the best at validation either. We've all got our own mental load going on, and it's easy to forget to validate our partner. Oh, how I would have loved for my husband to come home one day and say, "Wow. The teenager sure is being a b-hole today, isn't he?" Or, "You do such a good job with the kids. Thank you! Oh, and by the way you're pretty."

Or what about validation from society that without the work of stay-at-home moms, entire civilizations could fall apart? OK, maybe that's not true, but entire households for sure.

When you work outside the home, or even at home with an employer, you can often count on being part of a team and being talked to about your successes. Rewarded for the times you get it right. Or hearing words of praise when someone is proud of you. Stay-at-home moms don't always hear that. And when they do—in those rare occasions when the husband notices you did something like mopping or hanging up his laundry—it still doesn't feel like enough.

The act of being everything to everyone day in and day

out is draining, and frankly, it can easily lead down that slippery slope of depression.

The days when my kids were younger, I felt like I was on this hamster wheel. Clean up. Mess. Clean up. Mess. Clean up. Mess. And if my husband happened to come home during the Mess phase, I felt like I was failing. He never made me feel that way, but I often wondered why I couldn't just keep a clean house. What, like it's hard?

I know—seems like a joke to me now. *Now* I get it. *Now* I know why. But in those early stages of motherhood, it seemed like my whole life was just one giant task. Where was I amid all the laundry, dishes, and butt wiping? I was too busy being wrapped up in tasks that were never ending.

And no boss was patting me on the back to tell me I was doing a good job. (Although I hear that bosses rarely do that anyway.)

Besides, my bosses were little tyrannical toddlers and preschoolers who didn't care if I was having a bad day.

The babies sure weren't validating me either.

But then there were days when I did kick serious ass. I miraculously would accomplish a whole bunch and feel proud of my efforts. And often in those times, it would also go unnoticed. It's not to fault anyone here. It's just the nature of motherhood, right?

One day, I made a list of tasks I had done:

- I woke up early to make my birthday child French toast. I got three kids ready for school and out the door by myself,

- I headed to the gym, raced home to shower, and spent an hour putting all the stuff away all over my house.
- I spent my day pulling off the magic that has to happen for multiple birthday parties—making multiple trips to Target. (Rookie mistake. I now know that shopping for a picky tween must be done *with* the tween.)
- I baked a cake and did a little work on my computer, and somewhere in there I did three loads of laundry and let the cat in and out of the house approximately fifty-two times.
- I managed to get dinner started at 4:00 p.m. so I could run my child to his cello lesson (and sit through it so I can learn to play cello to help him practice) and then texted my oldest instructions on when dinner would be done so the house didn't burn down.

Let's not forget the fact I had also volunteered that week at the kids' school.

I loved my life back then when I was a stay-at-home mom. I felt privileged to be one.

All Those Tasks Can Lead to Depression

I didn't hear a "thank you" at all during that day. Not one. I didn't hear a "Wow, you cooked that amazing meal, baked a cake, *and* sat through a virtual cello lesson all at the same time?"

206

I didn't hear a "thank you" for clean laundry in their closets or for clean floors.

I didn't hear a "thank you" for the 9:00 p.m. grocery trip when I was bone tired to get the ice cream for the party the next day.

The truth is, I have good kids and a good husband. But it's depressing to be everything to everybody.

I looked back on that exhausting day and wondered if there was anything at all in that entire day I did for myself. I felt like a blur of a person—running to and from tasks.

That's how easy it is to slip into depression trying to complete tasks for everyone else in the family.

Spending nearly twenty-four hours a day as an unthanked workhorse would wear down even the most stable of us. (No pun intended.)

Yes, being a mom, whether you stay home or work, is a gift. It's a good life. But it's also not that hard to see why we crumble. Why we wonder what we're doing and how we became the personal assistant to everyone living under our roof.

The realization that I am the backbone of the whole operation is a heavy load.

If you're feeling depressed, here are some ideas:

Tell someone.
This will always be my advice when it comes to any mental illness: if your depression is making you think about suicide, call 988 (the Suicide and Crisis Lifeline) immediately. Also tell your partner and seek help from a professional.

Don't suffer depression alone. Tell a friend, family member, or doctor. Seek help. Let your partner know that validation would be nice.

Consider whether stay-at-home motherhood is for you.
A lot of women daydream of being able to stay home for kids until it happens. It's not for everyone, and there is no shame in that. But kudos to those who love it.

Make a list.
Finding the root of mental illness is always a good way to try to recover. Often, we need a professional to help us figure out if we have past childhood trauma or genetics, or if we just struggle being a stay-at-home mom. Consider making a list for yourself of what is making you unhappy in the moment. Dig deeper and ask the hard questions. Keep digging on your own, and if that doesn't work, seek a professional and uncover the root of your depression.

CHAPTER 22

Anxiety, the Evil Stepsister

Anxiety is like the sneaky evil stepsister to depression. You don't always realize she's the problem until she's ripped your dress apart on the night of the ball and stolen your pearls. She's usually the one whispering doubts and fears into your ear until you erupt in rage.

My mom used to tell me I was like this as a kid. I used to be the quiet antagonist to my much louder, sassier, more vocal sister. I would whisper things to ger her all riled up, making sure my mom couldn't hear. Then my sister would get so pissed at me for saying all these mean things Mom couldn't hear that she would hit, bite, or pinch me and I would start crying.

Initially, my sister would be the one getting in trouble (sorry, Linds) because she was the loud one who finally lashed out. But usually, the truth would come out that I was pushing all her buttons to get her in trouble. Before I knew it we were both getting punished.

I promise I've grown out of this.

Anxiety feels a lot like this to me. Something that is sneaky and tricky and then finally leaves you raging. *Why the hell am I so pissed off about another cup being taken out of the cupboard right after I just finished cleaning the kitchen?*

Anxiety Can Start Early in Your Parenting Journey

My anxiety has been a part of my parenting journey from the beginning. Postpartum anxiety is a thing, like postpartum depression. It's just not talked about as much. In many ways, postpartum anxiety robbed me from the joy of motherhood just as much as postpartum depression did.

I have memories of staring at my newborn's chest as she was soundly asleep with my mind racing. *Is she dead? Is she breathing? I should nap, too, but is she dead? Is she still breathing?*

When kids two and three came along, my anxieties manifested into things like obsessing over poopy diapers, sleep schedules, and rigid timelines to maintain some sense of control over my environment. It grew into irritation and anger with time because I wasn't always handling things well.

Anxiety Makes You Feel Robbed of Your Whole Motherhood Experience

A mom with anxiety struggles with a noisy brain full of what-ifs and worst-case scenarios along with annoying childhood TV songs like, "Paw Patrol. Paw Patrol. We'll meet you on the double!"

You stress about everything from whether your baby is getting enough sleep and eating enough to whether you're ruining your kids permanently and if one day they will write their own books about what it's like to have a parent with anxiety.

For me, big chunks of my life feel like a blur now. The years when I was untreated, I was in survival mode. I have these flashes of cute things my kids said and did. But so much of my experience during those years was trying to make it through the day without becoming the cracked egg with my insides oozing everywhere.

Anxiety Can Turn into Something Really Unhealthy

I could write a whole chapter about how anxiety can make you fixate on things and how if anxiety and depression are evil stepsisters, obsessive compulsivity is the evil twin.

It's not talked about as much because often OCD is seen as an illness having to do with cleanliness and germs; that's just one aspect of it. I see it more as a companion to anxiety. When your anxiety gets stuck in a loop, obsessiveness and compulsivity can be the result.

For me, this can look a lot like intrusive thoughts and hyperfocusing on a problem. While you might be thinking, "Gosh, it really sucks we all have the flu," I will take it to the next level with OCD. The worries about it will get stuck in a loop. This includes obsessing over cleanliness and germs in the case of getting the flu, but it can be obsessing over any aspect of parenting.

Maybe your child is struggling with learning to read and it's all you can think about it. That might be normal, but then you take it to the next step by making him read for three hours every day and neglecting your other kids' homework. Then you go one step further, and before you know it, you have dreams about reading with him and can't sleep because you're brainstorming ideas and you're making lists and charts and graphs to make him a better reader. It's all you can think about!

I touch briefly on OCD because, a lot like ADHD, it's one of those mental health issues that often goes undiagnosed. If you find yourself getting stuck in unhealthy thinking loops or compulsively doing certain steps or rituals, it might be time to talk to your doctor.

You Worry Anxiety Is Robbing Your Kids

When you live in fight-or-flight mode, like a mom with anxiety, you often have a harder time slowing down. As a result, you stress about whether your anxiety experience is going to rob your kids of a happy, healthy childhood.

You worry they will miss out or will inherit some of your fears.

Some days you feel crippled, frozen in the face of so many things to do. You wish things were different and will yourself to stop worrying and overthinking and overanalyzing. You can't help it. And you feel ashamed.

Anxious Moms Tend to Absorb All the Emotions

Do you feel pain when your kids do, and anger when they lash out?

Like me, you probably want to react differently, to be calm in your own mind and heart, but when the toddler is having a meltdown, before you know it, you're the one on the floor kicking and screaming. You long for an easygoing, relaxed personality and ultimately feel depressed for never being able to get there. Your shoulders are permanently affixed to your ears, and even a massage feels unrewarding.

I know these things because I am you. I have felt all these things in the darkest parts of my soul. I have yelled and sobbed and felt like my kids would be better off with someone else because I'm so tired.

Anxious Moms Try to Maintain the Ultimate Control

We've talked a lot in this book about controlling the uncontrollable. But when you have anxiety, you constantly live in this state of limbo.

Will the toddler listen to me today? How will I help my child with Common Core math homework when I have so much to do already? Do I need to beat up that kid who's teasing my second grader?

Anxious moms rarely go with the flow and they scare easily. No, seriously, my thirteen-year-old is constantly hiding around corners trying to scare me. It works every time. Just the other day, I was in the bathroom, and I thought the house was empty. But he had come home from school, realized I was in the bathroom, and was waiting outside to prank his mama for the one millionth time.

It's super fun to have an anxiety disorder and a child who loves to jump out and scare you.

The last time he did it, I noticed I had my fists balled up. I warned him if he kept that up, I might accidentally get so freaked out that I punch something.

Kids Still Love Their Anxious Moms

Kids will become compassionate and empathetic because of your example and maybe even because of your struggles.

Be honest with them when it's age appropriate. But tell them the truth. Tell them motherhood is harder than expected. Let them know you have always wanted to be the best mom and you often feel like a failure.

Kids don't see you under the umbrella of anxiety or depression. They just see Mama. They don't know the difference between a "normal" mom and an anxious mom.

And no matter how hard you try to convince yourself they would be better off without you, I can promise you they wouldn't. They want you. Only you.

What Should You Do If You Feel Like an Anxious Mom?

Consider these three steps:

Know that there is help.
People know how you feel, and better days actually are ahead even when it feels impossible to climb whatever mountain you're currently struggling to get over. Just like with depression, get help. Tell someone you're struggling.

Just hang on.
A big part of my journey living with anxiety is to remember to take it one moment at a time. If I look at the big picture, it can feel debilitating. Baby steps, as cliché as they sound, are the way to hang on when you feel overwhelmed by your anxiety. Sometimes you take it one day at a time, sometimes it's one hour at a time, and sometimes it's one minute at a time.

> Kids don't see you under the umbrella of anxiety or depression. They just see Mama.

Give yourself grace, and see yourself the way your child sees you.
My kid once told me I looked like a leprechaun when I came out of my room wearing a kelly-green cardigan. I thought I looked cute. Kids have no filter. They will take you at face value and usually accept you (unless you're wearing green). When you're older, they will see your faults, but that's OK

too. Talk to them about the flaws, and they are more likely to accept you for them.

I guarantee: our kids are glad to have us in their lives. Even if they don't always like us.

CHAPTER 23

Nice Seratonin, Where'd You Get It?

I cannot tell you the number of times I have opened up about mental illness while writing and gotten a tip that might help. Bless their hearts, people mean well. This happens in real life too. And I know they want the best for me. I know they want to give suggestions because it's human nature when we see suffering to want to fix it.

I will attest that when you are suffering from depression and anxiety, the last thing you want to hear is what worked for someone else. Why? Because more than likely you've already tried it. For all those who have found a cure for their anxiety and depression, I'm happy for you. I was offered tips like yoga, essential oils, dieting, meditation, and practicing more self-care. Those things may work for some, but when I tried them it was quite the opposite for me at the time.

I'm happy yoga worked for you. I really enjoy yoga when I can remember to do it. It calms me instead of making me realize there are muscles in my body that have never been used my entire life. And how do you possibly get your bodies in those positions? Kudos to you; mine doesn't bend that way.

I'm happy the essential oils did something for you. I've already mentioned how I diffused the hell out of some essential oils to cure everything from the common cold to that itch in the middle of my back I can never seem to reach. I love me some calming lavender, but I'm still an anxious mess after trying them all.

I'm happy you practiced more self-care. Ahh. The cure-all of self-care is important for anxiety and depression sufferers. The problem is, usually after self-care there's this pesky thing called mental illness that keeps sticking around after the margaritas and massages.

I'm happy for you if meditation does the trick. My mind is like Buddy from the movie *Elf*. Everything is in overdrive, and while it does help me focus a teensy bit, I still can't help getting distracted by a shiny thought floating into my brain.

I'm happy that adjusting the standard American diet worked for you and "*is the only way to live*." I'm happy you love kale chips. I love tortilla chips, so it's basically the same. I'm happy that juicing the organic carrots you grow in your sustainable, composted garden works for you. You keep doing you; it doesn't work the same for everyone.

I know you want me to trust you. You say, "Just try it."

"Just do a little deep breathing and open your mind a little more to your feelings and *feel* them."

I'm glad counting your blessings really helped you get through your rough patch. News flash: I totally have a house full of blessings. They have names, and I love them, and I still have anxiety and depression.

Truly. I'm happy for you if any of those things or a combination of them have helped or have cured you.

Let me tell you a little secret:

Some of us struggle with anxiety and depression no matter what we try.

Trust me. If you live with anxiety and depression, you have tried it all. I've gone on the long rage walks. I've sprinkled those oils, diffused them, rubbed them, and eaten them, and yet, when I last checked, yep—still depressed.

I love that four-square deep breathing exercise I learned in therapy years ago. Breathe in for four seconds. Hold for four seconds. Breathe out for four seconds. Repeat four times. It really helps calm me in the moment. No sarcasm. It does. But the funny thing about it: I still have anxiety.

I've done even crazier things—like when I went through a phase of religiously taking probiotics that cost me as much as a semester of college tuition. I've eaten special clay. Yes. Dirt. I've eaten dirt. Well, I mixed it with water, but it was still dirt water. And I would drink it. It was supposed to clean me out or help me out. The details are murky. Kind of like the color of the water. Green smoothies are yummy. But they don't cure my depression.

I have literally driven to the mountains near my home and taken in the sights and smells. Walked in the grass. Put my hands in the mud. Waded in the river.

Fun fact: I have taken ice-cold soaks in fifty-two-degree water. I was able to soak for five minutes straight. It was at a hot spring where you'd move from the super-hot spring to the cold spring and back again. I did sleep great that night. But yep, I've still got an anxiety disorder.

> **Green smoothies are yummy. But they don't cure my depression.**

For those of us who live with it daily, this isn't just a phase. This is a battle we fight every day within our minds. I still feel hopeful with each new suggestion and feel hopeless when that dark ugly stepsister named depression comes back.

The constant suggestions help us feel cared for, but they also make us feel like it's somehow our fault if yoga doesn't fix us.

Next time someone shares that she is struggling, sit with her in that dark place. Tell her you're glad she shared. Let her know you see her and hear her and don't know what to say—but you are there for her.

How You Can Help Someone You Know Who Is Struggling

Consider offering these two things:

Validation.

As I've mentioned before, we most want to hear you simply say, "I can't imagine. That sounds awful. Can I do anything?" We certainly don't need to be told we're doing it wrong or that our pill isn't the answer. We need validation that you see we're doing everything we can by taking that pill or going to therapy.

Empathy.

Just show up. Bring a coffee. Offer to take the kids for an outing. Give a hug. It's the simple acts of kindness that help us know you care and that you *see* us.

We are warriors fighting something many people don't believe is there. We don't want you to pretend it isn't there either. We want you to see us for who we are and be there. Let us know you get that it's hard.

To Medicate or Not: That Is a Question for Your Doctor

Years ago I made the decision to get on medication. It was not an easy choice, and I will be the first to say medication didn't "fix" mental illness. I had been going to therapy for about a year, desperate to avoid taking medication. I was on an antidepressant briefly after my second child was born, and it did help, but the side effects were awful. I had to stop taking it.

Fast forward several years, and I was in my therapist's office having a heart to heart. She knew I was trying to avoid medication, but I seemed to be swimming in circles in my sessions lately. Hung up on the same things. Having the same arguments with my husband. Dealing with the same fears and anxieties. I asked her if she were to diagnose me with something, what would she diagnose me with?

She gently told me she thought I suffered from generalized anxiety disorder (which I expected) and obsessive compulsive disorder (which I did not expect).

I hadn't shared with her about my obsessive hand washing or my obsession with worrying about my kids getting sick, so her diagnosis of OCD surprised me a bit.

I had a few quirks when I was a child that could fall under what I thought OCD looked like, but they had not come up in session. When I was younger I had to have things orderly before I could fall asleep, and I obsessively checked the door locks in the middle of the night almost every night.

I asked her why she thought I had OCD, and she told me it was because I seemed to obsess over conversations and thoughts more than the average person. And I have to tell you—it was like a light bulb clicked on. I felt instant relief.

Obsessing over conversations was kind of a superpower of mine. If you said something to me three weeks ago, more than likely you have already forgotten about it, right? However, there's a very solid chance I'm not only thinking about it but I've also charted out fifteen different ways I could have responded with more humor, sass, or kindness.

Usually, when people get "diagnosed" with something there is a lot of sadness, but this diagnosis actually made me happy.

I felt relief in that moment. Suddenly, so many things made sense, such as my rabbit-hole obsessions with everything from true crime murders I wanted to solve by listening to the podcast and reading the book. It was also why I couldn't sleep at night if something was left unsaid or unwritten. I finally had answers. I immediately followed her diagnosis by asking whether she thought I needed medication. She sat silent for a moment.

She did a typical neutral response that therapists are trained to do. You know, the one where they don't want to tell you what to do because that would be totally unethical, but they guide you to making the decision for yourself. In her gentle way, I knew she was telling me it was OK without telling me.

Being a people pleaser, I just wanted someone to give me permission. While she didn't exactly do that, she did tell me I had done some really hard work in therapy and "maybe it was time."

I didn't feel sad at that moment; I felt empowered.

What happened *after* I got that little bottle of pills was a different story.

I knew I needed the medication, but I felt numb as I went through the motions to get it. I was still hung up on the stigma of medicating myself even though my rational brain that studied psychology in college knew better.

Since my therapist couldn't prescribe anything for me, I went to my primary care doctor. It felt like an out-of-body experience to mutter those words *anxiety* and *depression* to yet another person. I halfway listened as the pharmacist talked to me about side effects and how to take it and when.

While the diagnosis had felt empowering, the idea of taking pills felt like failure. I brought the bottle home and left it on the counter. Every time I walked by, that bottle loomed like an admission of my failure. I told myself I'd take it in the morning, hoping the morning wouldn't come for about a million years. When I woke up the next day, I stared at that bottle. I only felt a slight sense of hope as I debated with myself.

Maybe I'm fine.

I'm not doing that bad, am I?

Why can't I do this on my own? I'm trying so hard.

It's not fair.

I felt a wave of emotions: anger, frustration, sadness. And I was tired. *So* tired. After staring at that bottle for what seemed like eternity, I took the pill.

I tried not to think about it until about an hour later when I felt nauseous and dizzy and was forced back to bed. *I must be getting sick.* Then I remembered. Oh yeah. The pill. These were the side effects. I regretted it instantly.

I felt horrible for the next three days. Dizzy, nauseous, and anxious about whether I made the right choice. Day after day, I took the pill, even though I didn't want to. I felt like a robot. I had finally admitted defeat.

Three months later, I was feeling better. Because if you can stick with it, the side effects do lessen over time. I felt stronger and hopeful, and happier most days. I felt like I was a calmer, better mom. I felt proud of the fact I obviously made the right choice.

I realize now taking that pill wasn't admitting defeat at all. It was evidence that I was being brave. It was admitting it's OK to need help. To be different. To fight for a better life. It was an admission I am willing to do what is right for me. Willing to fight for myself and my family. Willing to do hard things.

I'm stronger because of it.

So What Is the Cure for Mental Illness?

While I can't advise you on whether medication is the answer for you, or when you should get a therapist, I can share my experience so you can feel seen in your own struggle with whether to medicate or start therapy.

There is no easy cure. But we don't have to suffer alone. Professionals are willing to help guide us, and I can't emphasize enough how important it is to seek help.

Here are a few takeaways from my experience regarding "cures."

Finding the right medication takes time.
I've tried at least five different antidepressants over the years. None of them are perfect. They all have side effects. You can't get one prescription and think it will cure it all. It won't. Keep at it. Find a physician or a psychiatrist you trust, and advocate for yourself. What works for me might not work for you. We all have a different DNA.

Finding the right therapist feels like dating.
Therapists are amazing. But they are not all the same. They all have a different approach. I went to a lady once who was super focused on the deep breathing thing. While it helped, I found she didn't know how to deal with some of my other issues. We broke up.

I went to another therapist for a long time who loved group therapy. I loved it too until I found I still wanted to deal with some childhood trauma, and that wasn't her specialty. We broke up too.

Now I go to a therapist who really clicks with my personality. He gets my sense of dark humor and is helping me battle some really negative thinking patterns. We may not last forever, and that's OK.

If you're terrified of therapy, that's OK. It takes a while to find the one for you, but it's worth the time and energy.

Both therapy and medication can be temporary.
I shared my story about medication so you know it's OK if you don't want to medicate and you know that I fought it. It's important to remember both therapy and medication can be temporary things to help you. While mental illness is often a lifelong battle, you can switch things up as you are able. Try new methods, and talk with your doctor about how long you need to be on medication.

You know yourself best.
I'm no doctor, and I'm not a therapist. I often get messages asking me what I think and what I would do or even what kind of medication I'm on. You and your doctor can figure that out together. You know yourself best, and when you're struggling with mental illness, it's vital that you advocate for yourself to get the help you need. And if you don't feel like you have the energy to advocate, bring a friend or family member with you.

CHAPTER 24

Talk to Your Kids About Mental Illness

No matter how hard we try to do everything right, I'm sure our kids will one day sit across from a therapist and tell them something we did that scarred them for life. At least that is how I am envisioning it.

I hope they do seek out a therapist if they ever feel they need it. I'm 100 percent pro therapy. You get a therapist! You get a therapist! Everyone needs a therapist!

I don't hope they are screwed up from their childhoods, but everyone should go to therapy. The stigma around therapy is keeping us from getting the valuable skills and tools our children need.

As I've gone to therapy myself, I've been able to pass those skills down to my kids. I have shared tools to help them learn how to cope with hard things, discuss emotions, and become more self-aware.

My kids know how to use four-square breathing, go to their imagined happy place in their minds, and seek out calming techniques.

Life is hard, stressful, and messy. We go to school to learn how to do everything from writing a grammatically correct sentence to becoming a doctor.

We need those skills to survive in life, but guess what—we also need mental health skills to help us survive every day as human beings. We need help learning to become emotionally honest beings who are not afraid to work through hard things.

In therapy, I've learned a lot that has helped me improve myself, but I've also learned skills that have helped me survive life's really difficult challenges. Why wouldn't I want that for my kids some day?

What's a better skill than to teach our kids the importance of caring for their own mental health?

Dr. Samantha Rodman, a clinical psychologist, says she asks moms all the time if they would want their children to feel stressed like they feel stressed. They always say no.

So what's a better skill than to teach our kids the importance of caring for their own mental health? I'm still working on getting my kids to talk about their feelings. It's a lifelong work in progress.

Early Intervention and Awareness Can Make a Huge Difference

I had symptoms of mental illness as a child that were overlooked and unnoticed by my parents. Looking back, it would have been life changing to understand that some of the things I was feeling were because of my anxiety. It would have been a relief to know how to deep-breathe my way through a frustrating experience or tantrum rather than having a full-blown meltdown about nonexistent tornadoes in the sky. It would have been a miracle to have the skills to distract myself from incessant worrying.

It would have been helpful to know that I could count four things I can see, three things I can touch, two things I can hear, and one thing I can smell in order to escape a negative thinking pattern. It would have been a relief to recognize a panic attack for what it was instead of worrying that I was dying from a heart attack my sophomore year in college. That was not fun.

We all need skills, and therapy can help us through the mental health challenges that being human brings to us. We don't have to have a mental illness to need a little help now and then.

And therapy for kids can be really fun. If you could see the number of toys, gadgets, and fun sand boxes child therapists have in their offices, your kid might think he's going to play for an hour. Child therapy is fun. Yes, it's hard work too. I've watched one of my kiddos go through it. It is a beautiful gift to give a child.

Just as we need skills to know how to read and write, we need skills to know how to cope and thrive and love ourselves through this messy, difficult existence of life.

Talking About Mental Illness Can Change Lives

Ultimately, talking to our kids about mental health should be at the top of our list from the beginning of our parenting journey. As soon as we think they are emotionally mature enough to have the conversations, we should have them.

We probably shouldn't share too much too soon, and we definitely should avoid something like, "OK, so Mommy is a little crazy, and she has this anxiety disorder that makes her need medication and therapy and feel totally insecure about raising you." That sounds like a recipe for a kid's future therapy session if I've ever heard one.

But we can start young with our kids and have fun teaching them about how it's OK for them to have big feelings. We can name those feelings and validate them. We can parent our kids like we wish we had been parented.

We live in a different generation than our parents did. We are bringing the topic of mental health into the light so that more moms (parents) can talk openly about it and then educate their children about the importance of asking for help and talking through the hard stuff.

By having age-appropriate conversations with your kids about mental illness, you can also help them have empathy for you, for their peers, or even for themselves one day if they end up struggling with the same issues.

By Talking About Mental Health We Become a Safe Place for Our Kids

Engaging in conversations about mental health takes a lot of practice—consistently reiterating to your kids that their mental health is just as important as eating their veggies. To be honest, I don't think I was the greatest at this when my kids were young.

Society doesn't give parents the tools for raising a mentally stable baby. We hear the importance of teaching them how to eat healthy, walk, talk, go to school, learn math, and so on. But if we aren't emotionally mature, we're certainly going to have a more difficult time raising kids who are.

When COVID-19 was first introduced and everything was closing down, we looked at it as a super long summer. It felt like it was going to be fun to be together and get to skip out on some of the stress of the school year. When we were on lockdown, we had a good time playing games as a family and being together, and my kids started playing together in ways I hadn't seen in years. But as the days dragged on and reality set in, I, like many parents, saw a marked change in the mental health of each of my children.

It was the first time I started to panic that this pandemic would have long-lasting effects on their emotional well-being and social skills.

So we talked about it. A lot. I validated their feelings as much as I could, and while only time will tell how much of it helped, I did see a difference in the moments when they were validated in their feelings of sadness, fear, frustration, and loneliness.

We were talking about our feelings almost every day.

They knew it was OK to feel upset. What a gift that is to give to another person! To be able to allow a child to *feel*, be heard, and truly be himself or herself. And as parents we can do that for our kids.

That's special.

If you are a parent with a mental illness, you have a unique perspective to offer. You can emphasize for your kids the importance of being aware of their mental well-being. You can also offer techniques you have learned that will help them navigate the emotions they will face in their early years and later in life.

When to Talk to Your Kids About Mental Illness

So how do we know when it is appropriate to talk to our kids about our own mental illness? And why should we?

If our child broke a bone or had the flu, we would discuss it with him and help him through it. It should be no different with mental health issues.

The beauty of being able to share my own struggles with my kids is that we frequently have open discussions around feelings, failures, struggles, and stress. It gives them permission to have struggles and talk about them, but it also helps me explain why some days are harder for me than others. I can openly discuss when my stress levels are high or when I'm having a hard time functioning through anxiety and depression.

Society views some feelings as negative, but normalizing those feelings is the first step in talking about mental health with your kids. We can normalize feelings like anger when they're two years old and having a tantrum. We can normalize sadness when they are a toddler who doesn't get their way. We can start normalizing these things as soon as they can start carrying on a broken conversation with us.

As they grow older, you'll know how much more they can handle. I've had talks with my kids about mental health as they've heard about world events on the news and awful things like mass shootings.

Mental health is a huge part of our society, yet so often we leave it out of the conversation. Add it in. You'll know how much your kids can handle. And normalizing talking about mental illness may save their life or the life of one of their friends one day.

Don't Diminish Negative Feelings That Your Kids Express

When emotions are high, it's important that we don't slip into the trite sayings from childhood that our parents used. That's what was modeled for us, so that's likely our default response when dealing with stress with our kids. We might flippantly say something like, "Stop being so dramatic" instead of saying something validating like, "I can see this is hard for you." While I don't think we can always have enough Zen to stay calm like this with our kids, it's amazing the transformative change we see when we validate our children when we can.

It's OK to feel emotions. Even negative ones.

I heard "stop whining" a lot, when asking a question such as, "Why is this upsetting to you right now?" would have been a better option. That simple shift in phrasing might have helped me express the fear I was feeling in the moment or helped my parents see there was a reason behind the feeling. I wish I could have learned this earlier. Some kids are taught to feel shame around frustrating emotions. Angry emotions. Sad emotions. And instead of being able to communicate how they are feeling, they are often left feeling like no one understands. I worked hard to switch my verbiage and teach my children that it's OK to be disappointed and it's even OK to be mad at me.

The Culture of Toxic Positivity Can Easily Seep into Our Parenting

We can easily slip into the mistake of telling our kids it could be worse. Or at least they have food to eat. Or at least they have a friend even when that friend is being mean.

I am guilty of this. I have literally used the old saying that there are kids in Africa who don't get food and they better eat the dinner I made them. But how is this helpful? Kids don't have the perspective on life that we do. We want them to, but if we're being realistic, that's something that comes with time and life experience.

We should give our kids hope, yes, but life is hard. And

it's OK not to be OK for a little bit. Things will look up, but some situations that come our way are just sucky.

Coping Techniques Are Important Skills to Teach Kids

Most of us aren't born with the skills to tackle some of these big emotions. I know I wasn't. My skill set included hyper-focusing on perfectionism and kicking and screaming until someone paid attention to me. But as I have gotten older, I have learned through therapy that self-care is a skill and coping mechanisms are an important part of life.

Maybe you're one of those parents who doesn't have the financial resources to get your child therapy right now. That's OK. There is a plethora of information out there to help you and your kiddos learn to deal with big feelings and life's problems.

YouTube is a great resource. I've found excellent videos made for kids on yoga, meditation, emotions, and even more specific issues kids face such as ADHD, anxiety, and OCD. The more tools we have in our pockets when life throws us a curveball, the better we'll be able to handle disappoint-ment, anger, and all the hard things that happen.

Imagine raising kids who feel emotionally safe to express their feelings. By the time they are teenagers they will be facing big hard things. School adds pressure to their lives, but so does social media, social situations, fail-ure, and scary things like school shootings. Our kids face a lot today.

What Is Safe to Say to Our Kids?

I've been able to talk to all my kids about how my brain gets extra stressed. How I take medicine to help me. How I get overwhelmed easily. Kids need to see that's it's OK to have struggles, in order to accept the struggles in themselves. Maybe they are not working through a mental illness, but there's a good chance at some point in their life they will struggle with momentary or situational anxiety or depression.

If we can have an open dialogue about mental health in our homes, in a way children can understand, we are giving them permission to not be OK, and we are setting them up for a lifelong ability to manage their mental health in a way that is healthy for them.

CONCLUSION: LOOK AT YOU! YOU'RE DOING IT.

The takeaway I hope you get from this book is that we can't always "fix" the mental illness, the mental load, the toxic culture, or the lies we are expected to believe about motherhood.

The mother load is a real thing, and it never leaves us. Give me a mother, and I'll show you a woman who still worries about her kids, no matter how old they are.

Mothers are strong. We conquer the world when we have the energy, and we should give ourselves grace when we are at our max and just need a nap. Whether we're accomplishing tasks like crazy or just cuddling with our kids on the couch, we all love our kids, and that's the most important part of the parenting experience.

That's what our kids need.

We're not perfect, but motherhood was never meant to work that way. The overwhelm that comes from raising humans is a new normal that just comes with the territory. That's exactly what the mother load is.

We can spend time beating ourselves up for what we thought motherhood would be or what society told us it should be, or we can realize that motherhood lies somewhere in the messy middle.

Sometimes we make perfect meals full of veggies, and our kids eat them. Then other times we are scrambling, and we end up eating a mix of randoms from the fridge like string cheese and ketchup for dinner.

Sometimes we have cookies baked when they come home from school. Other times we are cranky and tired and make them do chores and yell a whole bunch until someone ends up crying.

Sometimes we are calm in the mornings before school and help them make their lunches. On occasion we grumpily bark orders and breathe a sigh of relief when they are finally out the door.

Some nights the bedtime routine is full of giggles and laughs and looking the other way when they are reading with a flashlight past their bedtime. Other times we rush through the routine, desperate for alone time.

We all feel like two different mothers sometimes: the one we imagined we would be and the one that we are.

But the truth lies somewhere in between.

We are not one or the other. We have good days and bad. We mess up and get it right.

We struggle some days and make it look effortless on other days. But the reality is that being perfect was never part of the deal we signed up for when we decided to take on the role of a mother. Perfection has always been out of reach.

The truth of beautiful motherhood lies in the real, raw, honest mess. It's in the gray areas where we are doing it less than perfectly (if not horribly). Beautiful motherhood is about raising our kids with love, and we have that in spades.

The mother load can trick us into thinking we're never measuring up. And our brains are never the same because that is the whole entire point of all of it. Motherhood has changed us. Our children have changed us. The weight of this job has changed our hearts and our minds. We love these humans into existence, we love them through this existence, and our minds and hearts are forever changed because of this parenting journey, whether we like it or not.

Author Jennifer Pastiloff said, "When I get to the end of my life, and I ask one final, 'What have I done?' let my answer be, 'I have done love.'"

At the expense of our pre-baby minds, we've loved the way we were intended to love. We may forever operate with this new, messy, often forgetful mind. We will always worry. We will screw up consistently. Yet we're doing the darn thing anyway to the best of our post-baby brain ability.

The mother load isn't about the weight of all the expectations we carry. It's about the change within each of us. It's a gift we've been given to carry this load with us forever.

And it's a beautiful load indeed.

ENDNOTES

1. Allison Daminger, "The Cognitive Dimension of Household Labor" in *American Sociological Review*, August 2019, 84(4), 609-633. https://journals.sagepub.com/doi/10.1177/0003122419859007

2. Lucia Ciciolla and Suniya S. Luthar, "Invisible Household Labor and Ramifications for Adjustment: Mothers as Captains of Households" in *Sex Roles*, October 2019, 81(7-8), 1-20. https://www.research-gate.net/publication/330847401_Invisible_Household_Labor_and_Ramifications_for_Adjustment_Mothers_as_Captains_of_Households

3. Kristalyn Salters-Pedneault, Ph.D., "What Is Emotional Validation?" in Verywell Mind, Nov. 14, 2022. https://www.verywellmind.com/what-is-emotional-validation-425336

4. Mitchell K. Bartholomew, Sarah J. Schoppe-Sullivan, Michael Glassman, "New Parents' Facebook Use at the Transition to Parenthood" in *Family Relations*, July 2012, 61(3),455-469.https://www.ncbi.nlm.nih.gov/pmc/articles/PMC3650729/

5. Secular Buddhism Podcast, Secular Buddhist Association.

6. Lena Groeger, "Happiness: Do we have a choice?" in ScienceLine, Jan. 28, 2011. https://scienceline.org/2011/01/happiness-do-we-have-a-choice/

7. Ibid.

8. Bonnie M. Le and Emily A. Impett, "The Costs of Suppressing Negative Emotions and Amplifying Positive

Emotions During Parental Caregiving" in *Personality and Social Psychology Bulletin*, March 2016, 42(3), 323–336. https://doi.org /10.1177/0146167216629122

ACKNOWLEDGEMENTS

The Mother Load is a book that's been weighing on my heart since the very first essay I ever wrote about motherhood and mental health. I never thought I would write it, because it's not easy to put all your deepest insecurities and flaws in print for the entire world to see. But I wrote it first and foremost for the women everywhere who share my same story.

To the many readers of my blog who encouraged me through their private messages of support and solidarity—thank you. I am forever grateful for women who are brave enough to speak out about the invisible battles they fight. And I'm forever grateful I got to write a book that is, I hope, a voice for the women who may never get to tell their own stories.

To Caroline and the entire team at Absolute Love Publishing—thank you for helping me believe that I could write any book at all. I will forever be grateful for your kind words, encouragement, and for taking a chance on a writer like me with Mom Life.

To Karen Longino—thank you for believing in me, this book, and this message. You helped me take a very rough draft I wrote in the middle of a pandemic and make it into something beautiful and worth reading.

To the team at Dexterity Publishing—you are shining examples of positivity and the friendliest people I've ever met. Thank you for helping me transform this book into something I'm proud of and hope my kids will read one day.

To my own therapists, who will not be named publicly because they are hard to get into and I don't want to share—thank you for normalizing, validating, encouraging, coaching, and doing all the things a good mental therapist does for a client. Because of you, I believe in the power of healing and found the courage to be who I was always meant to be.

To Robyn Gobbel, my own personal best friend therapist who is also actually a real therapist—thank you for being the kind of friend I can call after many months have passed and have two-hour conversations about all my existential problems. Somehow, I still walk away from those conversations feeling like I'm 1000% normal. Mostly.

To Mary Katherine Backstrom—thank you for being my best friend who is always willing to stick her neck out, pass along an amazing opportunity or connection, be my biggest cheerleader, and make me laugh until I pee my pants.

To Sara Farrell Baker, my funniest friend—thank you for being a shining example of why I should love myself. Without you, I wouldn't have the courage to be unapologetically me. You taught me that, and I will forever love you for it.

ACKNOWLEDGEMENTS

To Nicole Pilgrim—for 35-plus years you have always loved me exactly as I am—anxious, depressed, permed hair, and all. You will forever be a sister to me and thank you for always reading the nonsense I write.

To my sister Lindsey—you are the one I always want to call first about everything that happens. Through heaving sobs or crying laughter, you know me best. Thank you for being my person.

To my sister Paige—thank you for answering the phone even though you hate talking on the phone. Thank you for being an example of how to put one foot in front of the other and do the hard stuff anyway when life totally sucks. You're inspiring.

To my brother, Chris—you carried me through a really hard time in my life with encouraging words and an understanding ear. I am forever grateful.

To my parents—how do you thank someone in one or two sentences for giving you life and making you funny? You can't. But I love you and am grateful for all that you've given me.

To my girl—you made me a mom first and that's something special. Your budding feminism, confidence, and ability to be exactly who you are leaves me in awe. I love you.

To my amazing middle child—you teach me every day why it's important to laugh and serve others. Being your mom is a gift. I love you.

To the "baby" of the family—you exude joy and a love for life. You came into the world knowing exactly what you wanted out of life, and I hope all your dreams come true. I love you.

To Jon-David, the man who has stood by my side through the darkest times in my life and loves me no matter how many times I screw up—thank you for your support, love, encouragement, and acceptance of all the versions of me I've become over 20-plus years. You are more than I deserve. I love you.

ABOUT THE AUTHOR

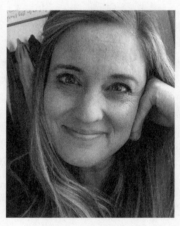 Meredith Ethington is an award-winning writer and author of the book *Mom Life*. She started writing on her popular blog, Perfection Pending, where her viral essays reach millions of struggling parents. She is also the co-founder and editor in chief of Filter Free Parents.

She lives in Salt Lake City, Utah, with her husband, three kids, and muppety dog, Millie. In her loads of spare time, she is studying to become a licensed mental health counselor.

She also has a cat, but honestly, she's a dog person.

To learn more about Meredith go to
perfectionpending.net.